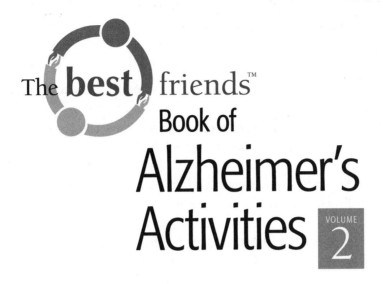

The **best** friends™
Book of
Alzheimer's
Activities

VOLUME
2

Additional titles available on Best Friends™ care practices

The Best Friends Book of Alzheimer's Activities
Volume One
Volume Two
by Virginia Bell, David Troxel, Tonya Cox & Robin Hamon

The Best Friends Approach to Alzheimer's Care
by Virginia Bell & David Troxel

Los Mejores Amigos en el Cuidado de Alzheimer
The Best Friends Approach to Alzheimer's Care (in Spanish)

The Best Friends Staff:
Building a Culture of Care in Alzheimer's Programs
by Virginia Bell & David Troxel

The Best Friends Daily Planner

Best Friends (DVD)
produced by the Greater Kentucky & Southern Indiana Alzheimer's Association

To order, contact Health Professions Press, Inc.
Post Office Box 10624 • Baltimore, MD 21285-0624
1-888-337-8808 • www.healthpropress.com

For additional information on the Best Friends™ approach,
visit **www.bestfriendsapproach.com**

———————

Have a question for a Best Friends™ Expert Leader?

Have a KNACK story or Best Friends™ Activity you would like to share?

Interested in training on the Best Friends™ Approach?

Interested in purchasing multiple copies of Best Friends™ books for your organization?

Email

bestfriends@healthpropress.com

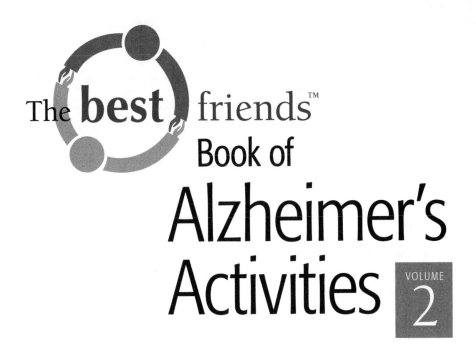

The **best** friends™

Book of
Alzheimer's
Activities

VOLUME 2

149 more ideas for creative engagements!

Virginia Bell, MSW

David Troxel, MPH

Tonya M. Cox, MSW

Robin Hamon, MSW

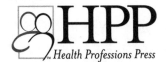

HPP
Health Professions Press

Baltimore • London • Sydney

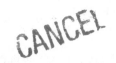

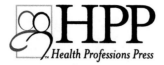

Health Professions Press, Inc.
Post Office Box 10624
Baltimore, MD 21285-0624
www.healthpropress.com

Second printing, December 2012
Third printing, December 2014

Typeset by A. W. Bennett, Inc.
Cover and interior designs by Erin Geoghegan.
Manufactured in the United States of America by Victor Graphics.

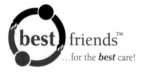

Best Friends™ is a trademark of Health Professions Press, Inc.

The following Best Friends™ titles are also available from Health Professions Press, Inc.:

The Best Friends Book of Alzheimer's Activities, Volume One

The Best Friends Approach to Alzheimer's Care

Los Mejores Amigos en el Cuidado de Alzheimer (*The Best Friends Approach to Alzheimer's Care* in Spanish)

The Best Friends Staff: Building a Culture of Care in Alzheimer's Programs

Best Friends (DVD)

To order, contact Health Professions Press, Inc., Post Office Box 10624, Baltimore, MD 21285-0624 (1-888-337-8808; www.healthpropress.com)

For more information about the Best Friends™ approach, visit www.bestfriendsapproach.com.

Library of Congress Cataloging-in-Publication Data
    The best friends book of Alzheimer's activities, volume two/ Virginia Bell . . . [et al.].
      p.   cm.
    ISBN-13: 978-1-932529-26-5 (papercover: alk. paper)
       1. Alzheimer's disease—Patients—Rehabilitation.   2. Alzheimer's disease—Patients—Long-term care.
3. Occupational therapy.   4. Recreational therapy.   I. Bell, Virginia
    RC523.B47 2004
    362.196'831—dc22   2004009606

British Library Cataloguing in Publication data are available from the British Library.

Contents

About the Authors

Virginia Bell, MSW, is Program Consultant for the Greater Kentucky and Southern Indiana Chapter of the Alzheimer's Association. She is founder of that association's award-winning "Best Friends" adult day center for *persons* with dementia. With David Troxel, she has co-authored numerous articles and books on dementia care. She has lectured about the Best Friends approach in more than 20 countries. She can be reached at bestfriendsvbell@aol.com.

David Troxel, MPH, most recently served as President and CEO of the Santa Barbara Alzheimer's Association. Today he is a consultant and speaker nationally and internationally for dementia care and long-term care programs. He has worked in the field of dementia care since 1986 and is a past executive board member of the American Public Health Association. He can be reached at bestfriendsdavid@aol.com.

Tonya M. Cox, MSW, is Vice President of Education and Programs for the Greater Kentucky and Southern Indiana Chapter of the Alzheimer's Association. She began working in dementia care in 1995 in the Best Friends adult day center developing and leading activities for *persons* with dementia. She also teaches and presents on activity programming and quality dementia care. She can be reached at ttincher@windstream.net.

Robin Hamon, MSW, is Caregiver Support Coordinator for the Alzheimer's Disease Center at the University of Kentucky Sanders-Brown Center on Aging. She worked with the local Alzheimer's Association for 11 years. During her tenure as program manager for the Best Friends adult day center, she developed a creative arts training program for staff and volunteers. She can be reached at adbestfriend@yahoo.com.

Read more about the authors at www.bestfriendsapproach.com.

Acknowledgments

My thanks to the staff of the Greater Kentucky and Southern Indiana Chapter of the Alzheimer's Association, especially those staff members and volunteers at the Best Friends adult day center who have for more than 23 years worked daily to provide creative activities for *persons* with dementia. I also thank my husband, Wayne, our children, and the "grands and greats" for always being supportive.

—Virginia Bell

I thank my many old and new friends working in the field of dementia care and the families I have met who are traveling the Alzheimer's journey. A special thank you to the staff and caregivers of Carlton Plaza in Sacramento who are best friends to my mother, Dorothy. Thanks, Dad, for the love you still give to Mom and me every day. I also want to acknowledge my partner, Ronald Spingarn, for his support.

—David Troxel

A special thank you to those who have given their time and creativity to developing programs in the Best Friends adult day center: Carla Guthrie, Laurie Dorough, April Stauffer, Lucy Summers, Becky Stapleton, and Fran Edwards. I also thank the Board of Directors and staff of the Greater Kentucky and Southern Indiana Chapter of the Alzheimer's Association. I thank my family and friends for their ongoing encouragement, especially my husband, Fred Cox, and my parents, Jim and Judy Tincher.

—Tonya M. Cox

Thank you to my mentors and dear friends, Virginia Bell, David Troxel, and Tonya Cox. I appreciate the pure joy and enthusiasm that we share for this work. Also thanks to my colleagues at the Sanders-Brown Center on Aging, Alzheimer's Disease Center at the University of Kentucky: Dr. William R. Markesbery, Dr. Charles D. Smith, Dr. Frederick Schmidt, Dr. Gregory Cooper, Dr. Gregory Jicha, Dr. Allison Caban Holt, Marie Smart, Alise Brickhouse, and Roberta Davis. Special thanks to Jeffery N. Howe for teaching me that it is possible to test a person's memory without sacrificing self-esteem, if it is done with a bold sense of humor, deep sensitivity, and a lot of love.

—Robin Hamon

We also thank the following individuals who contributed to this book: Peter Ashley, Christine Bryden, Rong-Chi Chen, Sharon Cohen, Jim Concotelli, Sydnee Conway, David Currier, Sylvia Fiano, Barbara Fister, Sally Fitch, Shirl Garnett, Marianne Smith Geula, Daphne Gormley, Rosemarie Harris, Charles "Chuck" Jackson, Lynn Jackson, Minnie Jim, Nancy Kahler, William "Bill" Keane, Julie Lamberti, Kathy Laurenhue,

Acknowledgments

Jeanne L. Lee, Cherry Liter, Mary Lockhart, Anne McAfee, Jean L. McInnis, James McKillop, Tracy Mobley, Darby Morhardt, Carole Mulliken, Harry Nelson, Tammie Nguyen, Theresa Nielsen, William O. Paulsell, Corinne Rovetti, Charles "Charley" Schneider, Samieh Shalash, Larry Sherman, Vinod Srivastava, Tap Steven, Kathleen "Mimi" Taylor, Richard Taylor, Marilyn Truscott, Patricia Wesley, Arthur Whitcomb, Amy Wise, Christa Yoakum, Ani Zsolnai, and Phil and Karen Zwicke.

Activity Title	Page	Arts	Exercise	Groups	Evenings	Late Dementia	One-to-One	Intergenerational	For Men	In-Home	Outings
A Day at the Races	95			•					•		•
A Day at the Spa	72		•	•							•
A Tree for All Seasons	138	•		•				•			
Accentuate the Positive	17				•		•				
An Old-Fashioned Tea	152	•		•	•		•			•	•
Astrology	104			•			•				
At the Close of the Day	196		•	•	•		•		•		
Autumn Leaves	100		•	•							•
Baha'i Faith	57			•	•	•	•			•	•
Balloon Prints	121	•	•	•	•	•	•	•	•	•	
Bean Mosaics	122	•		•	•		•	•		•	
Being an Advocate	220			•			•		•	•	
Blue Collage	120	•		•	•		•	•		•	
Bocce Ball	165		•	•				•	•		•
Bonjour or Hola!	29				•	•	•		•		
Bouquet Garni Herbs	150	•	•	•	•		•		•		
Bragging Rights	46			•		•			•		
Bread of Life	149		•	•	•					•	
Breathing for Health	77		•	•			•				
Buddhism	58			•	•	•	•			•	•
Bull's-Eye	164		•	•	•		•		•		
Celebration of Life	78	•	•	•		•			•		
Christianity	59	•		•	•	•	•			•	•
Color Wheel	176	•		•	•				•		
Confucianism	60			•	•	•	•				•
County Fair	167	•	•	•				•	•		
Crayon Melts	124	•		•			•	•		•	
Crazy for Cookbooks	154	•		•	•		•			•	
Creating a Web Page	222	•		•			•		•	•	
Daily Intentional Walking	69		•	•			•	•	•	•	•
Daisies	102			•			•	•			•
Decorating Pumpkins	180	•	•	•			•		•		•
Decoupage Eggs	125	•		•	•			•		•	
Did You Ever?	40			•	•		•	•	•		
Doing Nothing Is Doing Something	24			•	•	•	•		•		
Drawing and Painting to Music	193	•	•	•	•	•	•	•	•	•	
Dried Flowers	202	•		•	•		•			•	
Eggshell Picture Frames	131	•		•	•		•			•	
Embossing	126	•		•	•		•			•	
Evening Busy Room	197	•	•	•	•		•		•		
Fabric Flowers	127	•		•	•		•			•	
Famous Pairs	192			•	•					•	
Festive Wreaths	219	•		•			•		•	•	•

Activity Title	Page	Arts	Exercise	Groups	Evenings	Late Dementia	One-to-One	Intergenerational	For Men	In-Home	Outings
Flannel Boards	182	•		•			•	•		•	
Fun with Scarves	171		•	•		•					
Geometric Bookmarks	218	•		•	•		•	•	•	•	
Getting out of the "Doghouse"	211		•	•			•		•		•
Giant Crossword Puzzle	172			•	•				•		
Give Me Five!	107	•		•			•	•	•		
Group Dancing	75	•	•	•							
Guided Relaxation	80	•		•	•						
Hail to the Chief	98			•	•		•			•	
Halloween	105	•		•				•			
Handheld Fans	103			•							
Hands Up!	51	•	•	•			•	•			
Hanukkah: The Festival of Lights	108	•		•	•	•	•	•		•	
Happy Hour	187			•	•				•		•
Hieroglyphics	166	•			•		•		•	•	
Hinduism	61	•		•	•	•	•			•	•
Home-Canned Memories	47	•		•			•		•	•	
Homemade Ice Cream	156		•	•				•	•		
Horsing Around	106	•		•					•		•
Hungarian Pogacsa	158		•	•						•	
I Cast My Vote for . . .	174			•					•		
If the Shoe Fits	96			•					•	•	•
In My Merry Oldsmobile	175			•					•		
Indian Curry	144			•						•	
Invite Me to Read That	18				•		•	•		•	
Islam	62	•		•	•	•	•			•	•
Johnny Carson	203	•		•	•	•	•		•	•	
Journaling	28	•		•	•		•			•	
Judaism	63			•	•	•	•			•	•
Laughter Is the Best Medicine	74		•	•		•		•			
Leaf Polishing	179		•	•	•	•	•	•	•		
Life Is a Collage	38	•		•			•		•	•	
List Making	22			•	•		•		•	•	
Lunar New Year	89	•		•				•			
Lunch Bunch	216		•	•					•		•
Mail Call!	21		•		•	•	•		•	•	
Mailing a Card	221	•		•	•		•		•	•	
Making Bunzas	143		•	•	•					•	
Making Clay Tile Letters	123	•		•	•	•	•	•	•	•	
Making Sachet Bags	213	•	•	•		•				•	
Maple Harvest	109	•		•			•	•			•
Matching Squares	178			•	•		•	•	•	•	

Activity Title	Page	Arts	Exercise	Groups	Evenings	Late Dementia	One-to-One	Intergenerational	For Men	In-Home	Outings
Mona Lisa	111	•		•	•						
My Old Kentucky Home	41			•					•		•
Mysterious, Magical Moon	188			•	•		•		•	•	•
Native American Spirituality	64	•		•	•	•	•			•	•
Needlework	93	•	•	•	•		•			•	
Newspaper Art	132	•		•	•		•			•	
1950s	91	•		•							
Northern Lights	110	•		•	•			•	•		
Offering Gentle Help	25				•	•	•				
Oktoberfest	97	•		•					•		
Painting Tile Trivets	128	•		•	•		•	•		•	
Painting with String	135	•		•	•	•	•	•	•	•	
Partner Prints	129	•	•	•	•	•	•	•	•	•	
Partnering with a Museum	209	•	•	•					•		•
Pet Parade	212		•	•		•		•	•		
Photo Shoot	50	•		•							
Picture Memories	44	•					•			•	
Pie Fest	148			•							
Planning Group	163	•	•	•					•		•
Playing Cards	189			•	•				•	•	
Pressed Flowers	190	•	•	•	•		•	•	•	•	
Prompt Me with Dignity	27			•	•	•	•			•	
Pumpkin Seed Roasting	153			•			•	•		•	
Quilting	201	•	•	•	•		•			•	
Recycled Art	117	•		•	•		•			•	
Relaxation Hour	70	•	•	•	•	•	•				
Rubbings	130	•	•	•	•		•		•	•	
Sandpaper Tote Bags	217	•		•			•			•	•
Saved by the Bell	71	•	•	•				•			
Scavenger Hunt	173		•	•				•	•		
Skinny Books	214	•	•					•			•
Smile with Me	23				•	•	•			•	
Sorting with Meaning	191		•	•	•	•	•		•	•	
Spelling Bee	177			•	•		•	•	•		
Sponge Painting	136	•		•	•	•	•	•	•	•	
Spontaneous Style Show	26	•	•	•							
Spring Has Sprung	99		•	•							•
Stained Glass Windows	118	•		•	•		•			•	
Stick Design	133	•		•	•		•	•	•	•	
Strength Training	83		•	•			•		•	•	
Stop and Smell the Roses	76				•	•	•			•	•
Sweet as Honey	155			•		•	•		•	•	
Sweetheart Boulevard	49	•	•	•		•					
Tai Chi	82	•	•	•							•

Activity Title	Page	Arts	Exercise	Groups	Evenings	Late Dementia	One-to-One	Intergen-erational	For Men	In-Home	Outings
Talking About Art	199	•		•	•		•		•		
Tell Me a Story	168	•		•	•	•	•	•	•	•	
Tempting Tastes	151			•	•	•	•		•	•	
The Culture Bus	210	•	•	•					•		•
The Evening Meal	146			•	•					•	
The Price Is Right	170			•	•				•		
The Sound of Music	198	•		•	•	•					
Things I Like	36						•	•		•	
Think Inside the Box	20	•	•		•	•	•	•	•	•	
Thumbprints	42	•		•				•			
Timepieces	92			•					•		
Touring Mexico	101	•	•	•			•			•	•
Trivia with a Twist	200			•	•		•		•	•	
USA Today	43			•	•	•	•		•	•	
Wall Tapestry	137	•		•	•		•	•			
Watch This!	19				•	•	•		•	•	
Watercolor Techniques	134	•		•	•	•	•	•	•	•	
Weaving	194	•	•	•	•		•			•	
What I Like About You	48			•					•		
What We Have in Common	35						•				

*To persons with dementia,
who have taught us so much about quality dementia care.*

CHAPTER ONE

Introduction

Welcome to the second volume of *The Best Friends Book of Alzheimer's Activities*. The first volume, written for professionals and family caregivers, was published in 2004 and has enjoyed great success. We have been gratified that activities professionals have taken the Best Friends challenge to enhance their activity programming, be bold, try new ideas, and strive to give joy, interest, and dignity to those in their care.

An analogy that we used in the opening of the first book still has meaning. If you play baseball or softball and mis-hit the pitch when it comes at you, then you may hear an unpleasant-sounding thud and the ball won't go far. If you hit the ball just right, then you can almost hear the sweet spot and the ball will travel a long way. The goal of both Volumes One and Two is to help you hit a "home run" when it comes to activities: to hit the sweet spot.

Here is an example that was given to us by one activity director. Before he embraced the Best Friends philosophy, he would routinely do a crossword puzzle as a group activity. "It would drag on for about 30 minutes, kept alive only by my own energy and the interest of a few people." With the Best Friends approach, he now pauses along the way, discusses the words (e.g., "5 down is *ocean*. Can anyone name the oceans of the world?"), and encourages reminiscence. The crossword puzzle itself now becomes secondary; it's the being together that's important.

ABOUT VOLUME TWO

This book is meant to be a companion book to Volume One. It offers 149 new Best Friends activities. This book will be helpful to any family or professional caregiver of a *person* who has dementia and is at home, in an adult day center, or living in residential care.

We have repeated some of the basics of the Best Friends philosophy in this chapter for the reader's convenience, even though these are noted in the first activity book. Volume Two can stand alone.

We have kept the same format as Volume One: Activities are briefly described in a shaded box to the upper right or left of the page. "The Basics" describe what it takes to implement the activity. Then look for the Best Friends logo labeled "The Best Friends Way" for dozens of ideas about how to make the activity richer and more successful.

Although somewhat retitled, five chapter topics from Volume One are repeated, but with all new activities. These chapters are "Celebrating the Moment," "Adult Education," "Let's Create," "Games and Active Things to Do Together," and "In the Evening." We have given the readers new ideas on these topics because of "popular demand." These are the sections on which we have received the most reports of success!

In this field, ideas are constantly evolving. We are pleased, for example, to retitle the chapter "Recreating the Classroom Experience" from our first book to "Adult Education" to reflect feedback from many persons with early dementia that they want to keep learning and/or be exposed to new, stimulating ideas for as long as possible. The title "Adult Education" seems more respectful, hopeful, and consistent with new ideas that support "brain aerobics" and lifelong learning.

Five chapters are brand new: "Honoring the Life Story," "Religious and Spiritual Traditions," "Wellness," "In the Kitchen," and "Community Spirit." "Honoring the Life Story" offers activities that will not only celebrate the person's unique history but also create opportunities for staff members to learn new, helpful facts about persons who are in their care. "Religious and Spiritual Traditions" discusses eight different world religions or spiritual practices to offer ideas for keeping individuals connected with their faith. The chapter's activities can also be used for broader education and programs that celebrate our diversity. "Wellness" discusses activities that benefit us all, including persons with dementia. Practices such as relaxation, visualization, Tai Chi, breathing exercises, intentional walking, and others can bring enhanced emotional and physical well-being to persons with dementia and their caregivers. "In the Kitchen" is self-explanatory. We believe that food remains a great pleasure for many persons with dementia. The chapter offers some delicious recipes but also some sensory-rich experiences, including a number of activities with an ethnic twist. "Community Spirit" builds on our philosophy that persons with dementia often want to be involved in meaningful activities that help other people. The chapter offers ideas for keeping persons productive. It also suggests activities that can keep them in the community, whether it is going out to eat or going to a museum.

Once again, we offer a helpful grid of activities at the beginning of the book that summarizes how different activities can be used and also serves as a table of contents or easy way to find a particular activity.

A significant focus of Volume Two is to recognize the growing diversity in the United States as it is reflected in staff, clients, and families in our long-term care programs. This book includes many multicultural activities, including the material noted here on various world religions.

In Volume Two, activities are geared not only for persons who are in their 70s, 80s, and 90s but also for younger persons who are in their 50s and 60s and have dementia. The baby boomers are aging, and our programs will be challenged to meet the needs (and demands) of this unique generation.

For the first time, we are pleased also to include contributed activities from dementia programs in the United States and other countries. We solicited these activities via the Internet as well as through personal contacts and travels. We hope that you enjoy some of these activities from around the world.

Finally, Volume Two offers the unique perspective on activities from 21 persons who have dementia who have told us their fascinating stories. They have much to say about activities, as you will read in the following section.

PERSONS WITH EARLY DEMENTIA: THEIR VOICES HELPED SHAPE VOLUME TWO

One of the challenges of dementia is that the impact of the disease gradually prevents the person from doing many things that he or she once enjoyed. An engineer who loved his job may no longer be able to perform the needed calculations. A good cook may no longer be able to follow a complex recipe. Someone's weekly card game may go by the wayside if his or her friends are not patient or supportive.

In preparation for writing this book, we interviewed 21 individuals with early dementia by telephone, in-person visits, e-mail, and old-fashioned written correspondence. The group included many remarkably high-functioning persons; it was not intended to be a representative sample per se but a survey of advocates and individuals, many of whom have always led active lives.

The goal of our conversations was not only to learn more about their needs in terms of activities but also to get their advice and wisdom on how to help other *persons* with dementia, including those *persons* later in their illness.

Here are the results of our survey of *persons* with early dementia. The responses fall into seven categories, and we have highlighted several of the *persons* in each category. As James McKillop of Glasgow, Scotland, told us, "Don't believe people who think that *persons* with dementia cannot relearn an old skill or learn a new skill. I have met so many who dispel that fallacy!" Keep his words in mind as you read the next sections. It's time for a new way of thinking about activities for *persons* with dementia.

Persons with Dementia Advocate for Themselves and for Others with Dementia

Many health charities have their advocates—individuals with breast cancer or HIV/AIDS have long carried the torch for expanded research funding and services—sometimes rather vocally and contentiously, like any good advocate! In the dementia field, advocacy from *persons* is a relatively new phenomenon but a welcomed one. Many in our survey were involved in letter writing (and listserv advocacy), lecturing, writing articles and books, testifying to government committees, and media work. A number were challenging local and national Alzheimer's societies to be more responsive to *persons* with dementia, including board slots for *persons* with early dementia.

Richard Taylor, a psychologist from Texas, has written his story in a provocative and beautifully written book, *Alzheimer's from the Inside Out* (see Appendix 2). His campaign slogan for his advocacy work is "Enable me, re-enable me, and for God's sake, don't disable me!" Richard regularly e-mails a large listserv and has tirelessly challenged the national Alzheimer's Association to enhance programs for early dementia. He remains an active member of the U.S. Alzheimer's Association Dementia Advisory Committee. Richard says that his time to educate is short, and therefore he is pushing hard.

Peter Ashley of the United Kingdom has been a successful advocate for the rights of *persons* with dementia. At conferences and in interviews he says that he is "living with dementia, not dying with dementia," and has worked on European advanced directives and other projects. Peter is a well-known figure for many individuals who are active in Alzheimer's Disease International, and his work on various projects has added tremendous authenticity and quality.

Lynn Jackson is a nurse from British Columbia, Canada, and is the founding president of Dementia Advocacy and Support Network International (DASNI). She has inspired many with her words, such as these that she shared with us: "During my career, I felt my purpose in life was to help people. By contributing to DASNI and speaking out locally, nationally, and internationally, I again feel that I have a purpose in my life—that is to help those with early-stage dementia try to live their lives to the fullest."

Taking their message to heart, we believe that caregivers, day centers, and other programs can involve *persons* with dementia in advocacy efforts even later in the illness. Encourage them to speak up and speak out by writing postcards to elected officials, signing a petition, or assisting the local Alzheimer's Association at an event. Highlighting this idea, we have created the activity Being an Advocate in Chapter 11 (p. 220).

Persons with Dementia Continue to Help Others

If faced with a serious or terminal illness, many of us might want to spend the rest of our days on a beach or in more solitary activities. It was inspiring to note the altruism of many with whom we talked who are facing Alzheimer's disease or a related dementia. *Persons* who were interviewed in our group were determined to help others, including those with dementia as well as the world at large.

Sylvia Fiano, from North Carolina, is a retired registered nurse whose Alzheimer's disease was diagnosed in 1999 at the age of 46. Before her illness, she played tennis, wrote, listened to Motown music, and loved to dance. Now she tells us, "My brain will not let my feet be placed where I think they should go." She took up painting after her diagnosis. "My journey took me to the magical world of playing with acrylic paint as my medium." She now paints for creative release and regularly donates her paintings to be auctioned at special events that are sponsored by her local Alzheimer's Association.

Lawrence "Larry" Sherman is a retired attorney from Baltimore, Maryland. He enjoys writing and swapping stories about rural Appalachia, where he spent time as a young man. Music is his life. Today he plays his clarinet for other *persons* at his adult day program as well as for friends and family. He can announce the piece of music, tell you about it, and play it. "You remain alive as long as someone remembers you." Helping others gives Larry purpose and gives him faith that he will be remembered.

Charles "Charley" Schneider is a retired policeman and fireman from St. Louis, Missouri. He serves on the Dementia Advisory Committee of the U.S. Alzheimer's Association, which is made up of *persons* with early dementia. With Carole Mulliken, another contributor to this book, he developed a support group called Caring Together. That group offers both caregivers and *persons* with dementia an opportunity to meet together to discuss common concerns. He notes, "We have found the dynamics of us all being together very advantageous." In writing his book *Don't Bury Me* (see Appendix 2), he believed that a more positive perspective would be helpful and encouraging to others who are on the journey of dementia (see the appendix). We appreciate Charley's words about his work: "I have found that the more I apply myself to helping others, the better I feel myself."

Even late in the illness, *persons* with dementia gain satisfaction from helping others, be it sweeping a porch, offering a hug, or giving advice. It is reassuring that many retain this good nature and good will toward others throughout the journey of dementia. For more on this topic, see Chapter 11, "Community Spirit."

Persons with Dementia Have a Need to Stay Productive

Work has meaning beyond financial survival for many. Being productive can keep a *person* with dementia physically active and intellectually stimulated. It also builds self-esteem.

Jeanne L. Lee is from Hawaii and brings her optimistic "aloha" spirit to her current work as a writer and an entrepreneur. She has published a book about her experiences, *Just Love Me: My Life Turned Upside Down by Alzheimer's* (see Appendix 2), and has started a company called Alzheimer's Awareness & Prevention to spread the word. She serves as a support group leader and has been active in Internet support and chat groups: "Our chat group talks about everything from medical research to what we had for dinner. Some days we just answer questions of new people." She adds words with which many in our survey would agree: "Talking to people in the same boat is the MOST necessary part of my life, and what a group!"

Carole Mulliken, from Washington, Missouri, struggled after receiving a diagnosis of Alzheimer's disease. "Happiness hasn't come easy since I was diagnosed . . . what was left of my life after diagnosis was hours of an endless, sprawling vacuum." She began volunteering at a homeless shelter, serving meals, but she ended up in an environment where she regularly receives unconditional love: the local animal shelter.

"They (the animals) were lonely; they needed freedom, and they were desperate for companionship." She noted that the dogs were quite unruly, and she implemented a new technique with which she was familiar to calm the dogs. The shelter quickly adopted her strategy. We enjoyed her humor: "Through volunteerism, I have discovered how to keep my vacuum packed."

Marilyn Truscott of Ontario, Canada, enjoys many hobbies, including poetry writing, playing piano, gardening, knitting, needlepoint, and painting. She loved quilting but got to the point at which, in her own words, "I could not understand and follow patterns and instructions, couldn't picture inside my head how the pieces should fit and what was the right side and wrong side. . . . The sewing machine looked like an alien space machine at times. I had so much trouble using it." She learned to make accommodations: "I take my sewn quilt tops to quilters to put the batting and backing together. They machine-quilt the tops for me and attach the binding. This enables me to finish products by having others do what I cannot do. I do what I can when I can and try not to allow my projects or errors to tire or overwhelm me." Today she is involved in two quilting groups, but more important to her, she can give her beautiful quilts to her daughters for their homes.

Programs that care for *persons* with later stage dementia should take note of the importance of this section. We believe that many challenging behaviors stem from pure and simple boredom. Helping a *person* feel productive, even late in the illness (helping with simple chores such as folding towels, straightening pictures that hang on the wall, and brushing the dog) is meaningful and rewarding for most. The activities in this book are designed to help a *person* with dementia feel productive, particularly in Chapter 6, "Adult Education," and with the Planning Group in Chapter 9, "Games and Active Things to Do Together."

Persons with Dementia Embrace Their Creativity

Dr. Bruce Miller of the University of California–San Francisco Memory and Aging Center has suggested that *persons* with early Alzheimer's disease actually have a spike upward in their creativity. It was striking to us that almost half of the individuals with whom we spoke chose to involve themselves in creative pursuits. Some learned new skills, whereas others returned to old, long-neglected talents. It makes sense that in almost a Zen way, *persons* who are losing cognitive powers might find themselves more open to the creative, to the spiritual. This activity provides inner rewards and seems deeply satisfying, even therapeutic.

Daphne Gormley of Santa Barbara, California, received her diagnosis of Alzheimer's at 59 years of age. She tells us that she had a very positive response to the current dementia medications. She has thrown herself into her artwork, and many pieces depict her new life with dementia (including pictures of plaques and tangles and self-portraits). She uses water-soluble crayons and felt-tipped markers for her paintings. "Rather than limiting my artwork, my Alzheimer's seems to have unleashed a whole new area of creativity for me. One of the benefits of my art is that it provides me a way of communicating without words. The colors I use are colors I find to be joyous. . . . Alzheimer's has really taught me to concentrate on the things I can do, not on the things I can no longer do."

Sydnee Conway of Chicago was a flight attendant for American Airlines for 39 years. She now volunteers at Dignity Diner (meals for the homeless) and also volunteers with her trained therapy dogs. When she received her diagnosis, she decided to learn something new to fulfill a long interest in oil painting and took two 9-week classes on the subject. "A diagnosis of Alzheimer's does not mean you should lie down and die. It's been a wonderful opportunity for me to advance my knowledge and do something that, in spite of my condition, brings me great joy!"

Tap Steven lives in Santa Barbara, California, and has had a lifelong interest in poetry. After his diagnosis, he began writing again in earnest and even published a book of poems that was well received. He often reads his poems for various Alzheimer's Association events and is a beloved figure in Santa Barbara. One of his poems, written in 2002, entitled "It Is Not Promised" (see Appendix 2), shows an insight and a sensitivity into the disease. An excerpt follows:

> It is not promised that the shadows will not lengthen
> As the generous sun ignites the western sky.
> No one says that memory will strengthen
> As fleeting days give way to night hawk's cry.

Creativity should be encouraged by all dementia programs. To be successful, though, it is important for family and professional caregivers to work with *persons* with dementia to encourage them to be creative. It is the *process* that counts, not the *outcome*. There are many creative activities in Chapter 7, "Let's Create."

Persons with Dementia Find Support Through the Internet

Some of the *persons* whom we interviewed travel nationally and internationally (usually with assistance from a friend or family member). Others travel virtually via the World Wide Web! The Internet has created a global village that has benefited many *persons*, including many of the individuals with whom we spoke. For *persons* with dementia, the Internet encourages and allows connection and communication. It is also a place to have fun and learn. With local, regional, and international chat rooms and Internet bulletin boards, it is also a place for community. We have created an activity around the Internet, Creating a Web Page in Chapter 11 (p. 222).

Shirl Garnett of Perth, Australia, offered us the most surprising activity. She has a "virtual pet" on the Internet (www.neopets.com). She remarks, "Caring for a virtual pet means earning the 'neopoints' I need to buy food to feed my pets and groom them, including shampooing, conditioning, and brushing them. You can play games to earn the currency to buy the things you want. These games get me thinking and help my spatial concepts, numbers, spelling, and speed of decision." (This is also something that Shirl, who received her diagnosis at age 59, can share with her grandchildren!)

Mary Lockhart of Piedmont, Oklahoma, has used the Internet to create a personal Web site where she frequently writes in her journal. It is called Mary's Place and offers her journal as well as information about dementia and resources. Her online journaling is quite interesting. She tells us that the Web site journal helps her remember what kind of day she had. While not on the Web, Mary enjoys spending time with children, grandchildren, and great-grandchildren and motorhome trips with her husband. (Her Web site is listed in the appendix.)

Charles "Chuck" Jackson, whom you will meet in the next section, speaks of the power of the Internet: "I have gained awareness that there are connections between people who have never met through sharing and experiencing a disease together. Even though there are thousands of miles between us, we are still able to connect, understand, and help each other."

Persons with Dementia Enjoy Being in Nature

Being out-of-doors is spiritual, allows time for contemplation, is sensory, and is life-affirming for almost all of us. Sunshine gives us natural vitamin D and fights depression. No wonder so many with dementia have talked to us in this survey about the benefits of being in "Mother Nature."

Of interest is that many of the responders mentioned that they notice things in nature now that they have not seen before. Perhaps their dementia makes them more aware of their surroundings, with the ability to focus more on the moment than the rest of us, who are constantly multitasking.

Phil Zwicke of Santa Barbara, California, received his diagnosis at age 49. He had enjoyed a long relationship with the ocean and windsurfed on the Santa Barbara channel for many years. He continued this activity long into his illness, and it bolstered his self-esteem and raised his mood to be able to sail past dolphins and pelicans several times a week. With his wife Karen, he enjoyed painting abstract images using some of his memories of days on the ocean.

Charles "Chuck" Jackson of Oregon has thrown himself into creating beautiful photography and a spectacular garden that surrounds his home. He tells us, "Experiencing connection with the world around me—whether it is with people, plants, rocks, or animals—through all of my senses, [helps] the art and writing that I do. . . . Lately, I have been sculpting and casting leaves from my garden in concrete. I bend metal rods into stems and create garden flower stakes. I think that everything that I do is a triumph over the disease."

Harry Nelson received his diagnosis in his 60s and is a retired dentist and refugee from Hurricane Katrina. He moved to Lexington, Kentucky, and now spends much of his time out-of-doors enjoying nature, hiking, and camping. He has had to give up his passion for kayaking, finding it too challenging. At his adult day center, he participates in a walking club. He has a goal to see how many U.S. National Parks he can visit. We hope that he makes it to them all!

James McKillop of Glasgow, Scotland, reconnected to an old skill of photography. As mentioned in the beginning of this chapter, James not only relearned old skills but also learned new ones (e.g., using e-mail, mastering new cameras). He also told us that he used to take many family portraits. Now he is fascinated by the contrasts of nature and takes pictures of delicate flowers against a stormy background or butterflies amidst thistles. Despite his losses, there remains a keen instinct and intellect to his photography. His work has been shown in photography exhibitions, and he has published a book of photographs, *Opening Shutters—Opening Minds* (see the appendix).

For *persons* who are in late dementia and are residents of long-term care facilities, we think that it is imperative that they be encouraged to get out-of-doors on a regular basis. This keeps *persons* in touch with nature, elevates mood, and is life-affirming for all involved. A number of activities in this book celebrate the great outdoors, particularly in Chapter 5, "Wellness," and in Chapter 11, "Community Spirit."

Persons with Dementia Savor Time with Friends and Family

Today's family may consist of a traditional husband and wife, or it could be domestic partners, caring friends, or multigenerational households. Whatever one's definition of family, it is very important for *persons* with dementia to have a support network to provide that extra bit of help when needed and to help the *person* feel safe, secure, and valued. Many *persons* with dementia told us of their love for family and friends.

Arthur Whitcomb of Ventura, California, was a mental health counselor for 33 years before his diagnosis. He publishes on www.poetry.com. Much of his work revolves around his love for family, including a beautiful 2006 poem for his wife, Esther. An excerpt follows:

My heart beats the rhythm of
The setting sun, and my chest swelled
Like the waves
We face West, my love, my wife and me.

Although relationships often change over time, we appreciate Arthur's passion and embrace of romantic love in the beautiful poem about the two of them sitting on a beach at sunset.

Tracy Mobley of Elkland, Missouri, received a diagnosis of early-onset Alzheimer's disease at 38. Now 41, new dementia medications have helped. She has used this time to publish her first book, *Young Hope*, and more recently has completed a children's book with her 11-year-old son, Austin, entitled *I Remember When* (see Appendix 2). We think that it is especially meaningful that she has created a lasting legacy with her son. Years from now, he will be able to look back with pride and happy memories over writing a book with his mother.

Charley Schneider echoes the words of many in our survey in recognizing the contribution of his family to his ongoing health: "My wife, my children, and their families are the greatest source of pleasure and encouragement in my life, and spending time with them is so uplifting." He wrote his book for many reasons but primarily he "wanted my family to know that I am not bitter, scared, or resentful."

Christine Bryden (formerly Christine Boden) is a trailblazing woman who was one of the first to speak and write about the life of *persons* who receive a diagnosis of dementia at a young age in *Dancing with Dementia* (see Appendix 2). She tells us that, for her, the unstructured activities and times are often the most important: "The memorable moments have been those when someone has stayed alongside me with words of encouragement. It is those times when we feel connected with another human being, when we feel valued and loved for who we are, not measured in some way for how we perform; that we can be comforted and supported by the knowledge that we retain our human dignity and sense of self in relation to others."

As we think about activities for *persons* with dementia, it is important to note that so many programs are only about structured activities, when what *persons* with dementia often most crave is that moment of connection or intimacy that can just take a few minutes! For more on this, see Chapter 3, "Honoring the Life Story."

BEING REMEMBERED

We thank the previously named individuals for their contributions to our work and for their ideas that will inspire so many others. As Larry Sherman said in his interview, "You remain alive as long as someone remembers you." We hope that their contributions to this book will keep their names, ideas, and contributions alive for many years to come.

ABOUT THE BEST FRIENDS MODEL

Simply put, the Best Friends philosophy is that *persons* with dementia need a "Best Friend," someone who will be empathic and supportive and travel the journey with them. Specific parts of the model include the following:

- **Understanding what it is like to have Alzheimer's disease or related dementias:** Best Friends accept that behaviors that seem strange or unreasonable become quite understandable when you know their origins. The Best Friends approach suggests that knowing the cause of a behavior allows you to give *persons* what they need, when they need it, whether it is reassurance, physical contact, or a comment or gesture that helps them "save face."
- **Learning the basics of dementia:** Best Friends do not need to become experts at research, but it is important to have a good understanding of the basics of Alzheimer's disease and dementia. Keep yourself and staff up to date by attending conferences, reading new books, and visiting reputable Web sites.
- **Strength-based assessment:** Best Friends focus on what a *person* can still do, instead of the things that a *person* with dementia can no longer do. Does the *person* still enjoy music, reading the newspaper, or taking walks? Don't aim too low with your activity programming; this robs the *person* of dignity. If you aim too high, however, you will invite frustration and failure.
- **Effective communication:** Best Friends communicate well and know the "dos" and "don'ts" of communicating with *persons* with dementia. Practicing active listening, speaking clearly and with simple sentences, giving compliments, and asking opinions help us better connect to *persons* and build a successful activity program. Each activity in this book includes conversation starters that will be useful for caregivers who are hoping to get the most out of an activity.

For more information about the Best Friends model, visit www.bestfriendsapproach.com or refer to this book's companion volumes, *The Best Friends Approach to Alzheimer's Care* (1996), *The Best Friends Staff: Building a Culture of Care in Alzheimer's Programs* (2002), and *The Best Friends Book of Alzheimer's Activities, Volume One* (2004). All are published by Health Professions Press. Also, a book for family caregivers is available called *A Dignified Life: The Best friends Approach to Alzheimer's Care* (Health Communications, Inc., 2002).

DEVELOPING KNACK

Knack is the goal of the Best Friends philosophy. It is defined as "the art of doing difficult things with ease" or "clever tricks and strategies."

When you follow the activities in this book, you take an everyday activity and add extra value and pizzazz. You can turn a meal into an opportunity for sharing life stories, a walk into time to explore nature, brushing teeth into an opportunity to tell a joke, and an art activity into one that touches the spirit. Doing these activities and finding success also help staff understand, learn, and live the knack.

HOW TO USE THIS BOOK

When we began writing this book, we asked activities staff what they needed most. Almost all said that they want a book that they can "grab and go." This book meets this need with 149 activities that can be used for one-to-one activities; group activities; and activities for 1 hour, 1 day, or even a whole "theme" week.

While these activities can be adapted for almost anyone, they are aimed primarily at *persons* who are in the middle stages or course of Alzheimer's disease or related dementias. These individuals generally cannot initiate activities on their own. They need a caregiver's or staff member's help to stay connected to activities, but once they begin, they can successfully participate. The activities in this book can be used in residential, in-home, and day center environments.

Each Activity Page

We start every activity page with a brief introduction or summary in a gray, shaded box that discusses the activity in general and makes some specific remarks about how the activity particularly benefits *persons* with dementia. Read this gray box first.

The Basics

The Basics section contains the ingredients to pull together the activity. The ingredients might include supplies that you need for an arts project (e.g., paint, paper, tools) or a caregiving technique (e.g., find a quiet place, bring up a favorite topic of the person). Also in this section are Variations (another activity or list of activities that are based on a variation of a theme discussed on the page) and Tips (general tips to help the activity run smoothly).

The Best Friends Way

This is where an everyday activity becomes an activity that is done with knack. Our suggestions are grouped in categories that range from ways to extend an activity using music or the arts to emphasizing particular spiritual or sensory benefits. We encourage staff members who do the activities to sample the ideas in this section so that they can learn the process of converting everyday "humdrum" activities into ones with flair. We suggest many ways to do this; you will certainly come up with more on your own.

Life Story: Recognizing each *person's* history and experiences is a fundamental part of the Best Friends model. To deliver quality care, we need to individualize care whenever possible. In an activity environment, this can include designing activities around a *person's* past or present. It can also include acknowledging the life stories of individual members of a group, including their attitudes, values, traditions, and history.

The Arts: Activities are enriched when tied to the arts. This can include connecting an activity to a widely known painting, reading a poem aloud, playing classical music, or admiring a sculpture. Many of the activities also involve participating in the arts, something that can be done as actual artists or as armchair critics.

Music: Music should be woven into as many activities as possible because it remains a source of joy for many *persons* with dementia. Even after they have lost language skills, individuals' memories of old songs are often intact. We suggest songs to sing, most of which are widely known. If you don't know the lyrics, then search the Internet for sites that contain song lyrics, or purchase song books.

Exercise: We take note of any opportunities for stretching, walking, or other physical activities that benefit the *person* and staff member. It is so valuable to keep the body moving because exercise builds strength, relieves boredom, and helps use up nervous energy. It is intriguing that recent research suggests that exercise may slow the progression of dementia.

Humor: We sometimes forget just how enjoyable laughter can be. Whether the source of humor is a joke, a humorous anecdote, or even a timely smile or gesture, laughter is a beneficial and therapeutic addition to almost any activity.

Old Sayings: Experienced staff members know that reciting old sayings is a favorite thing for *persons* to do. Therefore, throughout the book we suggest old sayings appropriate to the activity. Although many memories fade, many *persons* with dementia can still complete old sayings, such as "an apple a day keeps the doctor away," and find joy and satisfaction in discussing its meaning.

Old Skills: *Persons* may recall learned motor skills or other skills that they have practiced in their life. We encourage activities that help *persons* practice these old skills, be it flipping a pancake, spinning a wooden top, or sweeping the floor. Successfully engaging in old skills builds a *person's* self-esteem and confidence.

Sensory: The best activities involve the five senses of taste, touch, smell, hearing, and seeing. For example, peeling an orange can be a rich sensory treat and can be an activity in and of itself! Sensory activities are particularly enjoyable for *persons* with dementia and are also helpful for *persons* with advanced dementia who may not be able to participate in group activities.

Spirituality: Best Friends activities touch on the spiritual—whether it be acknowledging and embracing a *person's* religious faith or celebrating the *person's* spiritual nature. Spirituality often expresses itself through the arts, through music, or through long-held life values such as helping others. Although not everyone is part of a religious faith, we believe that everyone has a spirit that can be touched.

Early Dementia: In this section, we note whether the activity or part of the activity may be particularly helpful for *persons* with early dementia. Although definitions of stages vary, for the purpose of this book, it includes individuals who have awareness of their situation and can initiate and do activities on their own or with minimal supervision.

Late Dementia: Activity programs sometimes neglect *persons* with late dementia. Their ability to participate is limited, but they enjoy being in a joyful environment. Activities that involve the senses, such as music and touch, are particularly appropriate.

Conversation: Each activity concludes with some conversation starters that are tied to the activity. Many staff members have told us that this part of Volume One was particularly helpful, because it gave them the words and more confidence to get something started with the *person* in their care.

An ounce of prevention . . . : We assume that staff have basic competencies and common sense. Proper supervision is important in dementia care. At the bottom of some activities, we offer a few words of caution. Do not let this comment dissuade you from trying an activity; just use the tip to ensure that the activity is safe.

The Best Friends Book of Alzheimer's Activities, Volume Two, provides a rich source of ideas. We encourage you to train staff in activities by picking one or two from this book to do together in a staff meeting. You can also use this book as a springboard for new ideas. Get together a team and an easel and butcher-paper pad. Pick a chapter and work through the activities together. Which ones would be best for your program? Can your group come up with a dozen new ideas? Families can do similar work by going through the book together and picking activities to try at home.

A FEW WORDS ABOUT THE INTERNET

We recommend that Internet access be made available to activities staff to plan their programs. Search engines such as Yahoo and Google are rich sources of song lyrics, trivia, and pictures. We also like online encyclopedias, such as Wikipedia. For more about the Internet, see Volume One or your local junior high school student!

SOME NOTES ABOUT THIS BOOK

In this book, we describe individuals who have dementia with an italicized word *person*. We hope that this reminds the reader that the *person* with dementia, despite his or her cognitive losses, is just like the rest of us, with all of the same feelings and needs. This is also more economical for the reader than constantly saying "the person with dementia."

We use the word *dementia* in the book to describe any *person* with Alzheimer's disease or a related dementia. Alzheimer's disease remains the most common form of dementia, but we are learning more every day about the other dementias. The ideas in this book generally will work with any adult with cognitive loss, whatever his or her specific diagnosis.

We have written this book assuming that the reader has some basic knowledge about dementia and some common sense about activities. Some activities books that we have reviewed describe the "how to" or "basics" of the activity in such detail as to be almost laughable (e.g., pick up the song book, open the song book, find the right page in the song book, and sing). We hope that we hit the right balance for the reader in being clear with our instructions but not ridiculous.

One principle of *person*-centered care that we first wrote about in *The Best Friends Approach to Alzheimer's Care* is that every individual with dementia seems to follow his or her own unique course of illness. Some *persons* lose language skills early; others remain surprisingly verbal. Some *persons* advance rapidly, and others live with dementia for 20 years. We continue to believe that "if you've met one *person* with Alzheimer's disease, you've met one *person* with Alzheimer's disease." This suggests that it is even more important to individualize our approach to activities, give the *person* as much choice as possible, and remember that there is a *person* beneath the cloak of dementia, one who deserves our very best care.

CHAPTER TWO

Celebrating the Moment

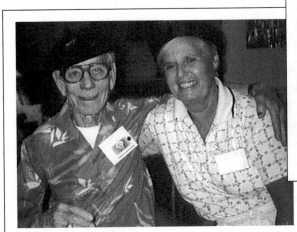

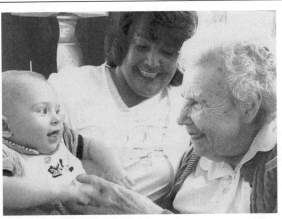

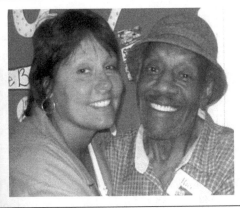

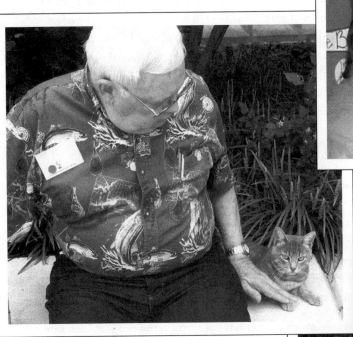

Celebrating the Moment

Over the years, we have often been asked, "What is the difference between a *good* dementia care program and a *great* dementia care program?" If we had to name just one thing, it would be this: Staff members in a great dementia care program go the extra mile. They take the 30 seconds to be a little less task-oriented and a bit more person-centered. They give the friendly hugs, use the life stories of *persons* with dementia to make a connection, smile, make eye contact, or tell a funny joke.

Doing the activities in this chapter builds bonds of friendship and trust. Positive relationships improve personal care routines, enhance dignity, and increase morale for *persons* with dementia, staff, and family members.

Christine Bryden, who has early dementia and was mentioned in Chapter 1, supports the importance of moment-to-moment times. Recall her eloquent words: "The memorable moments have been those when someone has stayed alongside me with words of encouragement. It is those times when we feel connected with another human being, when we feel valued and loved for who we are, not measured in some way for how we perform, that we can be comforted and supported by the knowledge that we retain our human dignity and sense of self in relation to others."

What Christine needs and wants doesn't cost any money, doesn't require an elaborate supply closet, and doesn't take much time! It takes staff with what we call "the knack," or the art of doing difficult things with ease.

Persons with dementia in many ways are in *the present moment*. Many have forgotten much of their past and may not be able to plan or visualize their future. They are often looking at their world more carefully than the rest of us; they can see the red robin in the tree or stop, slow down, and listen to a beautiful song.

Daily life is not always planned and structured. Even the best activity calendar cannot take into account weather, a *person's* mood that day, staff changes, or unexpected events. Because of this, spending some time with the activities in this chapter will help fill in the gaps and create as many meaningful moments as possible during the day.

We draw your attention to a few specific activities in this chapter:

Bonjour or Hola! (p. 29) is a fun activity that celebrates the heritage of many in the program and offers a simple learning exercise. Greeting a *person* in his or her native language creates a nostalgic moment.

Theme boxes, discussed in an activity playfully called Think Inside the Box (p. 20), are something that many programs have but don't use to their full potential. Read the activity in full to learn how to maximize the use of these boxes for reminiscence and conversation.

Many of the activities lend themselves to one-to-one environments, such as Smile with Me (p. 23), Mail Call! (p. 21), and List Making (p. 22). Others work best in groups, such as Spontaneous Style Show (p. 26) and the ambitious Journaling (p. 28).

A key to implementing this chapter is to recognize that a good program has moments of success throughout the day. When you string these moments together, like pearls on a string, something beautiful happens: Your whole activity program begins to shine!

In this chapter, as in the rest of the book, we introduce the topic, give a few basics, encourage you to tie the activity to the *person's* life story, demonstrate the activity's benefit in a number of categories, and then bring it all together with some conversation starters. At the end of some activities, we offer a few words of caution under "An ounce of prevention . . ." (with an umbrella icon). We hope that this chapter not only encourages celebration of the moment with *persons* but also with each other!

Tips for staff training: One way to encourage staff to think about celebrating the moment is to brainstorm creatively things that you can do in 30 seconds or less. At a staff meeting, divide the room in two groups and ask each group to come up with as many 30-second activities as the participants can. The winning team gets a prize. Share some of the answers (e.g., showing a picture, smelling perfume, giving a pat on the back, straightening a crooked picture on the wall).

You can also choose a few activities in this chapter to do at a staff meeting. At first, staff may grumble, but then they often will sit back and enjoy something different. Make the point that if they enjoyed this activity, then *persons* in their care will, too.

CHAPTER TWO ACTIVITIES

The Basics ————————————

Creating lists of positive qualities or attributes can be a small-group project or a one-to-one activity any time of the day.

One-to-one: Look for the ways in which a *person* makes a positive difference in themselves and others. The list could include the way one greets another, the smiles given, the sensitive way in which one pushes another in a wheelchair, participates with enthusiasm in a group session, or helps with the resident dog. You can also focus on past contributions made to the community or to other family members. Give affirming compliments and praise throughout the day to help *persons* feel connected.

Small-group session: Make a game out of Accentuate the Positive by talking about one positive characteristic of each *person.* Use a flipchart to record the positive qualities, and allow time for each *person* to bask in the acknowledgment.

Training Tip: Staff should model, accentuating the positive by looking for what staff members are doing right so that they in turn can do the same for *persons* who are in their care.

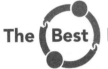

The (Best) Friends Way ————————————

Life Story: What in the *person's* life story is most valued by him or her: career, work ethic, family, religious faith, military service, community interests, or travels?

The Arts: Praise a *person* for his or her creativity in the field of art. Be specific by saying, "I like the way you are blending those colors to make a fall landscape" or "Your poetry always tells a story."

Music: Look up the lyrics to "Accentuate the Positive, Eliminate the Negative" and sing the song.

Humor: In your use of this activity, remind everyone of the power of humor as a positive for the giver and the receiver.

Early Dementia: *Persons* thrive on positive, authentic affirmations.

Late Dementia: The tone of positive language can be detected even when words are difficult to understand.

Conversation: Take the time: "Alvin, I appreciate your help with the music session. I like the way you made sure that each *person* had a program." "Thank you, Ollie, for laughing at my corny joke." Note: "Josephine, you saved a chair for me. I love sitting next to you." Compliment: "Stanley, you make me feel good whenever I am with you."

Accentuate the Positive

Affirmation: We all have needed a good dose of it since birth. *Persons* with dementia often cannot be self-affirming—as a result of loss of insight, language, and memory—and need affirmation in small doses from us all through the day.

An ounce of prevention . . .

Take the time to look for the positives, and always be genuine with each positive affirmation. A person may be astute in catching you when you overdo his or her strength or ability. Be aware that some persons embarrass easily; tread lightly.

Invite Me to Read That

Reading aloud not only is reading words for others to hear but is also a way to express one's personality. Many *persons* with dementia delight in being able to use this old skill of reading aloud, fine-tuned through the years.

The Basics

Begin collecting books that have short, descriptive passages about adult subjects, such as books with brief descriptions of countries, states and presidents of the United States, celebrations, flowers, birds, and oceans. Brainstorm all the ways to invite *persons* to read aloud. For example, when a topic is being discussed, ask someone to read facts about the subject for the group. Have the information typed on an individual card so as not to be confusing. He or she can share interesting stories from a newspaper, celebrate a birthday with a poem read aloud, or greet or introduce a guest by reading a prepared message.

Variations: As a community project, partner with a school class to read aloud to the students and encourage the students to reverse the idea and read aloud to others. Read aloud selections at a "This Is Your Life" celebration (see Volume One, This Is Your Life, p. 104).

The 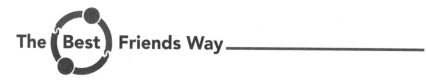 Best Friends Way

Life Story: Invite the *person* to read aloud from his or her hometown newspaper, alumni magazine, or horoscope. Some *persons* are writers and have published books and articles and may be pleased to share some of their own work with the group. Did anyone participate in a Reading for the Blind program? Who has read for a religious service or community service? Does anyone remember when he or she learned to read? Has someone memorized a favorite poem, or would he or she read it to the group in a poetry reading?

The Arts: Read aloud something about the composers or artists being discussed that day.

Old Skill: *Persons* have read aloud since they first learned to read.

Spirituality: Ask a *person* to read aloud a passage from a sacred text (see Chapter 4, "Religious and Spiritual Traditions").

Early Dementia: A *person* can often excel in this area and can feel a sense of fulfillment in the process. Take advantage of every opportunity to ask a *person* who enjoys reading aloud to help with any selections that can be shared with the group.

Conversation: Give a compliment: "Zeke, you read the greeting with a lot of enthusiasm." Ask for an opinion: "Rose, did you get nervous as a little girl when the teacher asked you to read aloud?" Ask for help: "Chuck, I left my glasses at home. Will you help me read this paragraph aloud for the group?" "Larry, would you read one of the poems you've written?"

An ounce of prevention . . .

With dementia, old skills such as reading diminish over time; this activity will not be appropriate for everybody.

The Basics

It takes only a few minutes to demonstrate a skill or show off a talent. Take time to blow up a balloon, demonstrate a magic trick, twirl a hula hoop, do a jumping jack, dance a jig, stand on your head, turn a cartwheel, spin a top, make a funny face, blow a bubble, play with a yo-yo, draw a picture, clown around, or play a tune on a harmonica.

Training Tip: This activity is so simple that it easily can be overlooked. Brainstorm with the staff all the small ways in which members can perform to the delight of *persons* with dementia. Some staff members may have a special "trick" that they would delight in sharing. Challenge them to come up with a list of 30 things that can be done in 30 seconds or less.

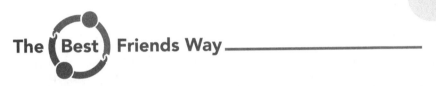

The (Best) Friends Way

Life Story: Use the life story for clues as to what the *person* may enjoy watching. When a *person* seems to enjoy a certain trick or tune, make note of this.

The Arts: This is a good way to incorporate music, dance, poetry, or painting into the day's schedule in a spontaneous way.

Exercise: Entice a *person* to move to music with you, or take a brief walk.

Humor: When doing this activity ham it up, brag, and be a bit silly. It can be fun for all when you show off a hidden talent, like balancing a quarter on your nose.

Old Skills: By watching others, a *person* may be reminded of one of his or her old skills, such as spinning a top or blowing bubbles.

Sensory: This activity can be full of motion, laughter, colors, sounds, aromas, and give-and-take conversation to prime the senses.

Spirituality: Taking the time to have fun with another helps the *person* feel that someone cares. A *person* may not remember the details of a spontaneous activity, but he or she may remember the joy at the moment, and that joy can carry over into the remainder of the day.

Conversation: Ask for assistance: "Tonya, would you give me a hand with this rope?" Notice the body movements: "Ralph, I loved the way you tapped your foot when I played that tune." Seek an opinion: "Helmut, would you like to play with this yo-yo?" "Sabrina, would you like to try on this grass skirt? I think you are a hula dancer at heart."

Think Inside the Box

Theme boxes can be used to provide immediate conversation topics and fun things to do together. *Persons* with dementia will enjoy looking at the items that spark old memories, and the boxes make great "grab and go" activities.

The Basics _____

Fill small- or medium-sized plastic boxes with items related to a particular theme. The items should be fun to explore and spark discussion on the particular topic. Themes can be nearly anything. A few ideas are gardening, office work, weddings, cars, travel, and sports. For example, a gardening theme box can include seed packets, gloves, a spade, seed catalogs, clay pots, a straw hat, a watering can, and a trowel.

Training Tip: Many programs have theme boxes that gather dust on the shelves. Be sure to train staff how to use them, and encourage their use!

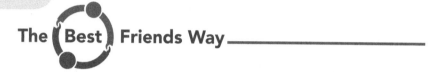

The (Best) Friends Way _____

Life Story: Design theme boxes around the interests and life story of the *person*. Consider putting personal memorabilia in the boxes. Create a theme box of individual keepsakes.

The Arts: Include index cards with instructions for art projects related to the theme. Label or decorate the outside of the boxes to reflect the theme.

Music: Include a list of songs related to the theme, such as lullabies for babies or love songs for weddings.

Exercise: Build in some kind of physical activity in each box whenever possible (e.g., a ball to toss in the sports box).

Humor: Create a laughing theme box that includes funny pictures, jokes, and silly mementos.

Old Sayings: Include a list of old sayings related to the theme, such as "a green thumb" for gardening. Create a theme box on old sayings.

Sensory: Be sure to find things that will stimulate all of the senses, such as baby lotion for a box on babies, textured fabric for a box on quilting, dried herbs for a box on gardening, or a colorful lure for a box on fishing.

Spirituality: Create a theme box around a particular religious tradition or spiritual practice.

Early Dementia: Invite the *person* to help you brainstorm a list of items to go into theme boxes or ideas for different categories.

Late Dementia: The tactile stimulation of items in a theme box can be very good for *persons* who are in late dementia.

Conversation: For a theme box related to fishing, ask: "Jim, did you use this kind of lure when you went fishing?" For a theme box for gardening, ask: "Which pair of gloves would work better when we're pruning the roses?" "Which tool would work well for this job?" For a theme box related to babies, ask, "Millie, did your mother make your clothes when you were a little girl?"

The Basics _____

- Mail, including advertising circulars, catalogs, holiday cards, junk mail, or letters from friends and family.
- Letter opener (optional).

Caregivers can work with the *person* to appropriately sort mail, taking care that bills or other important letters are not lost. Go through each piece of mail and discuss the content, colorful graphics or pictures, or price of the item being offered. Decide together whether to "keep or toss."

Tip: Encourage *persons* with dementia to read aloud items of interest.

Variation: Check e-mails daily if the *person* receives correspondence in this manner, and provide help as needed.

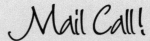

Mail Call!

Most of us set aside a time in the day when we take a few minutes to sort through our mail. *Persons* with dementia like to continue past rituals and respond well to having a routine and a purposeful task such as this one.

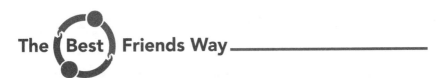

The (Best) Friends Way _____

Life Story: Did that *person* always review the mail and make the decisions about it, or did he or she leave it for someone else? Was the mail delivered at home or to a post office? Did he or she enjoy writing postcards while on vacation? Order a magazine subscription for a publication with many colorful photographs, based on the *person's* hobbies or interests.

Music: Sing the old Beatles song "P.S. I Love You," Elvis's "Return to Sender," or the Supremes' "Mr. Postman."

Humor: Make a point to look for funny pictures or ads in the mail.

Old Skills: Ask the *person* to stack together the newspapers or mail to be tossed for recycling. Using a letter opener is an old skill for many.

Sensory: As the *person* holds the pile of mail, he or she can enjoy the colors of envelopes and smell of newsprint, notice the unique handwriting of any hand-addressed letters, and clip and save colorful postage stamps.

Spirituality: Keep in contact by letters or e-mail with loved ones who live far away so that they may stay involved in the *person's* life.

Early Dementia: The *person* may file the letters that he or she does not want to throw away in a filing drawer or an accordion folder marked "letters from friends," "postcards," or "Judy's birthday cards."

Late Dementia: Read aloud a letter from the *person's* son or daughter.

Conversation: Assign a simple task: "Juanita, will you look for a grocery ad? Let's find out what is on sale before we go to the store tomorrow." Reflect on an old saying: "John, what do you think of the old saying about mail that neither rain, nor sleet, nor snow keeps postmen from their appointed rounds?"

An ounce of prevention . . .

Use common sense. If he or she is stressed by bills, do not include them in the activity. Be wary of bogus charity solicitations.

List Making

We all make lists of many kinds, from groceries that we need to buy to telephone calls that we need to make. This activity involves individuals or groups of *persons* with dementia in the task of making lists, an old skill that has meaning for many.

The Basics

- Paper
- Pencil or pen
- Dry-erase board or flipchart (optional)

Decide on a topic, such as tools I have used, books I have read, states/countries I have visited, flowers I have grown, places I want to go, varieties of apples, parts of a car, who is coming to a party, birds that I like, or days to celebrate. Write down everything you can think of that fits. This activity can be done one-to-one or in a group with a dry-erase board or flipchart with everyone contributing to the list.

Tip: Gently restate the title of the list and the items already on the list if the *person* forgets in the middle of the conversation.

The 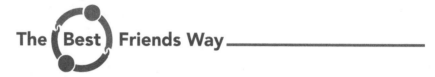 Best Friends Way

Life Story: Make lists that are based on what you know of the *person's* interests, for example, a list of tools for a retired carpenter. Did he or she always have a "to do" list to organize the day?

Music: List favorite songs, or list the songs in a song book. Sing together, "He's making a list and checking it twice. Gonna find out who's naughty or nice. Santa Claus is coming to town."

Humor: Make lists of famous comedians.

Old Skills: Writing things down is an old skill that many will enjoy, as is thumbing through lists of family members and addresses.

Sensory: It can feel good to hold the pencil and paper and be in control of writing down the words.

Spirituality: Make a list of holy cities or sacred places (*persons* from different religions will make different lists). List the books in the Bible. List the most beautiful places on Earth. List the most precious sounds you can hear.

Early Dementia: Making lists is one of the first ways of coping with memory loss. Make a "to do" list for that day.

Late Dementia: Make lists that require knowledge from long-term memory, such as holidays, fruits, vintage cars, or games played as a child.

Conversation: Invite participation: "Harry, we have six of the Seven Wonders of the World on our list. Will you let me read them to you so that you can help us find the one we have missed?" Reminisce: "Grayson, did you make a list of the gifts you wanted Santa to bring you?" Laugh together: "Minnie, did you keep a list of all of your boyfriends?"

The Basics —————————————

Collect from magazines photographs that feature smiling people. Pass around and discuss, or make a collage of smiles of people of all ages and cultures. List all of the things that can bring a smile to a *person*, such as telling funny stories and jokes, looking at funny pictures, engaging in teasing with a humorous twist, or clowning around. Ask a *person* to choose another in the group to give a smile. Ask the *person* who received the smile how he or she felt.

Variation: Use a digital camera to take pictures of *persons* smiling; print and pass around, or put on a bulletin board or into a collage.

Smile with Me

A smile is universally recognized and can instantly communicate that all is well. Giving a genuine smile to *persons* with dementia may be the best activity of their day.

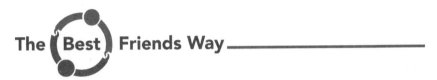

The (Best) Friends Way —————————————

Life Story: Some *persons* may have grown up in families who not only smiled contagiously but also laughed a lot. Mine the life stories for humorous stories that can be told and retold for many smiles.

The Arts: Read Ella Wilcox's poem "Smile and the World Smiles with You." Look at a picture of the Mona Lisa, and talk about her smile.

Music: Sing the song "Smile" by Charlie Chaplin.

Exercise: A smile exercises many muscles in the face. Any exercise goes better with a smile.

Humor: Have a contest to see who can give the best smile. Look at pictures of animals that seem to be smiling.

Old Sayings: "Smile, you're on 'Candid Camera.' " "She has a million-dollar smile." "Grinning like a Cheshire cat."

Sensory: Seeing a smile instantly communicates a positive note, and some *persons* will carress your cheek as if to feel it.

Spirituality: A *person* is automatically drawn to a smile, helping him or her feel connected and known.

Late Dementia: *Persons* can understand and respond to a smile, sometimes in a subtle way through the twinkle in their eyes.

Conversation: With a smile: "Cesar, would you please hold this pan for me?" Give a compliment: "Binnie, your smile makes me smile, too." Provide a question to think about: "Lloyd, do you think dogs smile?" Ask while viewing a picture of a *person* smiling: "Why do you think this *person* is smiling?" Ponder: "Is a grin the same as a smile?"

Doing Nothing Is Doing Something

Sometimes we prefer not to be engaged in an active way. *Persons* with dementia often want quiet time or need extra rest but still benefit from our presence and support.

The Basics _____

Sit quietly beside a *person*. Friendship can be so comforting that there is often no need for words. Be available and occasionally show some sign of affection, such as a smile, a soft pat, or a gentle hug. Your presence is a gift by itself. Ask the *person* to sit beside you while you work at your desk, at your computer, or at any task that is conducive to having a friend beside you. Be sensitive to cues from the *person* that he or she would like to begin a conversation.

The 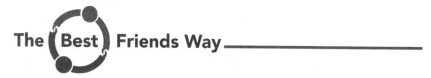 Best Friends Way _____

Life Story: Understand whether the *person* may have always been quiet and self-contained or the "life of the party" and always on the go. Did the *person* ever engage in solitary pursuits, such as fishing or reading?

The Arts: A favorite poem read or quoted together can connect us to each other.

Music: Background music, humming, or singing a familiar song may be appreciated.

Humor: Joke about being "couch potatoes."

Old Sayings: "Down time." "Having more time than money!"

Sensory: Nothing feels quite like a caring friend sitting very close.

Spirituality: A favorite prayer, a sacred writing, or a song may be the way to close a time of sitting together.

Early Dementia: Give a *person* your undivided attention, through your gentle presence, as he or she processes whatever is happening.

Late Dementia: A *person* may not be able to interact but may respond to a warm body beside him or her or a soft stroke on the hand. It can also be comforting simply to sit in the room with a *person* while writing or reading.

Conversation: The communication may need to be mostly nonverbal. Gain eye contact and give your best smile. Put your arm around the *person* and whisper: "Roman, I love you." Hum a favorite tune while squeezing Delores's hand. Connect: "Joyce, I feel better when you are sitting beside me." Ask for a kiss: "Otto, could you give me a kiss right here on my cheek?" Ask in a light-hearted way: "Would you rather vacation on a beach for a week and do nothing, or see seven countries in seven days?"

An ounce of prevention . . .

Do not assume that a person who occasionally wants to be inactive always wants to be inactive.

The Basics

There are many ways to help a *person,* but the offer should be concrete. Examples include helping someone tuck in his or her shirt, turn a page, go to his or her room, tie his or her shoe, change positions, or find a purse. Look for signs that *persons* give when they need help, such as calling out, wandering, or showing pained expressions, restlessness or agitation.

Training Tip: Help staff members become more sensitive to the many ways in which they can help a *person* who cannot initiate asking others for help. Have them brainstorm all of the ways in which *persons* may need help and are unable to ask for assistance. Ask the staff to note any difference that can be seen in the *person's* overall well-being after the training session, and discuss the outcome.

Most of us readily ask for help when we are in need of some assistance. This activity offers tips for recognizing when *persons* with dementia need help and how to offer it with a gentle touch.

The (Best) Friends Way

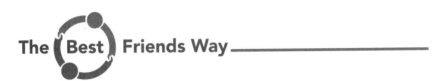

Life Story: Knowing a *person's* life story helps caregivers become better detectives in reading the signs that someone needs help. A devout Catholic who holds up her hand and fingers into the air might be asking for her rosary. A woman who had always been a meticulous housekeeper might be agitated at the overflowing wastebasket in the hallway.

Music: Music can be so consoling to *persons,* but often they cannot initiate turning on a radio or CD player to listen to their favorite music. A helping hand can make the difference in a *person's* day.

Humor: Ease a situation with humor: [While someone is having trouble eating], "That Jell-O must be on roller skates. Let me help you."

Old Sayings: "Two hands are better than one." "A helping hand."

Spirituality: Being there for the *person* is a spiritual act for both the *person* with dementia and the care provider.

Early Dementia: *Persons* can sometimes articulate their needs and yet be very sensitive when they have to ask for help.

Late Dementia: Checking for ways to help is especially important in late dementia, when *persons* have more difficulty communicating their needs.

Conversation: Place the blame on something else: "Marjorie, that sleeve is not made right. Here, let me help you." Add some humor: "Looks like a dog has chewed this page. No wonder it is hard to turn. I can help you." Help the *person* who is undressing inappropriately save face: "Let me help you put your slacks back on. I want you to come with me to hear the music program that is about to start on the patio."

Spontaneous Style Show

Who is not pleased to show off a new blouse or a new shirt? It can be the beginning of a spontaneous style show. With encouragement, a *person* can display a favorite piece of clothing.

The Basics

This activity needs no props. It may begin when a *person* has something new or looks especially pretty in her pale green sweater. She may be asked whether she would like to stand and model her new sweater or walk around like a fashion model. This idea can be expanded by asking each *person* to note something special that he or she is wearing and if he or she would like to show off this special article of clothing. The style show can include a special cap or hat; shoes or boots; purses; and any jewelry, such as a ring, watch, bracelet, or necklace. Take time after each *person* has modeled his or her outfit to mention something about each *person's* life.

Variation: Bring in clothing catalogs or fashion magazines to peruse to create a dream wardrobe.

The 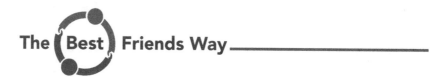 Best Friends Way

Life Story: Does the *person* like to shop? What is the *person's* favorite color? How did he or she dress while employed? Did he or she wear a uniform or wear a hat? Did she ever participate in a Junior League or charity fashion show?

The Arts: Take digital pictures of some of the residents, highlighting their outfits or accessories (e.g., purses, earrings, necklaces), and create a collage art project with them.

Music: Play background music while each *person* is highlighted. Sing, "Here she is, Miss America."

Exercise: Enjoy the art of movement as some *persons* dramatically participate in the show. Invite *persons* to walk around and model something special to them.

Humor: You might find a funny hat or cap for someone to try on for laughs. You can kid and announce a *person* as "Mr. or Mrs. America."

Old Sayings: "Pretty is as pretty does." "Clothes make the man."

Old Skills: "Showing off" is an old skill often enjoyed.

Sensory: The colors of clothing and the sounds of laughter can be a moment of sensory awareness for the *person*.

Late Dementia: Compliments are appreciated long into the disease.

Conversation: Speculate: "Chuck, what does the saying 'dressed to the nines' mean?" Joke and kid: "Orien, did you ever think of being a model?" Ask for help with your wardrobe: "Lillian, would you go shopping with me? I love your style." Have a debate: "Ladies, do you think the world treats you better when you are all dressed up?"

An ounce of prevention . . .

Be sensitive to those who may be in wheelchairs, and assist them to model with flair.

The Basics _____

A prompt is a verbal or physical motion that is intended to help a *person* start or continue an action. Prompting fills a moment of uncertainty with an idea or a place to start.

For caregivers, it is often challenging to strike the right balance between helping too much and not helping enough. The goal is to maintain dignity and self-respect by enabling the *person* to continue using his or her remaining skills, physical and cognitive, as long as possible and helping in a sensitive way when help is needed. Prompting can help fill the gap between what a *person* can do for him- or herself and the help needed.

Positive approaches to prompting include observing and assessing the part of the skill that is intact and which part is missing, using eye contact, calling the *person* by his or her preferred name, demonstrating cheerful body language, taking one step at a time if needed, and always helping the *person* "save face." This is also a good time to connect with the *person* by using other facts and experiences from his or her life story to assist with your prompt.

Training Tip: Organize an in-service session for staff around the skills of prompting. Use role-play to demonstrate the wrong way, and ask the staff for suggestions for a better way.

Submitted by Bill Keane, Long-Term Care Consultant, Chicago, IL.

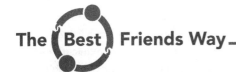

The (Best) Friends Way _____

Life Story: Is he or she extra sensitive about needing help or does the *person* welcome a helping hand? Is the *person* proud or independent? Has he or she had a strong work ethic that can be used to encourage participation in a meaningful activity?

Exercise: Remember to let each *person* do as much for him- or herself as possible. Each movement helps keep the muscles flexible.

Humor: Prompting sets the stage for the use of humor. You can laugh together at some of the situations when you are trying to help, and admit at times, "I'm clumsy as a clown!"

Early Dementia: Ask the *person* how he or she wants help.

Late Dementia: Nonverbal prompting, such as gestures, may be understood better. You may need to prompt using hand over hand. Remember to prompt one step at a time.

Conversation: Be aware: "Grace, maybe this soup spoon will work better. Now you can finish your delicious lunch." Ask to help: "Nicholas, this peg may be too big to fit in that hole. May I help you with this smaller one?" Blame something else: "Nellie, the sleeve of your sweater is hiding. May I help you?" Prompt softly: "Thank you for drying that dish. Set it down on the counter next to the sink."

Prompt Me with Dignity

When we are at a loss for words, a verbal prompt from a friend or a colleague can save the day. *Persons* with dementia also appreciate a thoughtful prompt as long as it is done with knack and protects dignity.

An ounce of prevention . . .

Keep your prompts discreet so as not to cause embarrassment when in group settings.

Journaling

Many of us have kept a journal or diary at times during our life. Journaling can be meaningful for *persons* with dementia if a caregiver is there to encourage and support this effort.

The Basics

- Journal or small notebook for each *person*
- Pens

Gather *persons* around a table with the journals and pens. Begin by talking about the concept of writing down thoughts and ideas in a journal. Present a topic to discuss and encourage *persons* to express their ideas on the subject. After the discussion, ask whether they would like to write their ideas in their journal. If they need assistance, then they can share their ideas with a staff member or volunteer for journaling on their behalf. Topics can be anything that the group would like to discuss. Examples include the *person's* favorite vacation, type of food, childhood memories, career or careers, and pets.

After writing in the journal, date the entry and keep the journal for future entries. This will be a meaningful gift to the family when the journal is completed. This activity can be done once or on a regular basis.

Submitted by Anne McAfee, Director of Risk Management, Elmcroft Assisted Living, Louisville, KY.

The 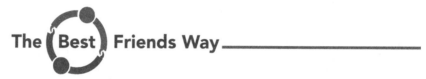 Best Friends Way

Life Story: Use the life story to identify potential discussion topics. Has the *person* enjoyed keeping a diary or journaling? Did the *person* write for a living, either in his or her business or as someone involved in journalism or communications? Was he or she an avid reader, perhaps reading biographies or autobiographies?

The Arts: Personalize the journals by asking the *person* to decorate the outside covers.

Music: Play soft instrumental background music. Ask the *person* to record his or her thoughts about a particular musical piece.

Exercise: Writing exercises the hands, wrist, and arms.

Humor: Ask the *person* to write about something funny that has happened in his or her life.

Old Sayings: "The pen is mightier than the sword." "A penny for your thoughts."

Old Skills: Writing and spelling tap into old skills.

Early Dementia: Journaling can be an excellent outlet for continued expression, thoughts, and feelings about the changes that *persons* are experiencing.

Conversation: Brag about someone: "Did you know that Matt was the editor of his college newspaper? He's quite a writer." Encourage: "Judy, what are a few words to describe your love of cooking?" or "Reverend James, write down how you felt after giving a successful sermon."

An ounce of prevention . . .

This activity is not for everyone, but it is an example of ambitious activity programming that is worth trying. In a group environment, involve a number of caregivers to give more personalized support.

The Basics _____

Each language has a familiar greeting that becomes a significant part of each *person's* tradition. In English, most of us respond to a simple "hello" or "hi." Find out what that greeting is for each *person* in the group, and teach the greeting to all those who relate to the *person* throughout the day. It will build self-esteem for the *person* and also be fun for the staff to learn greetings in other languages. The staff may be from a different tradition and can help with the teaching. Following are a few examples of familiar greetings in other languages (for a list of greetings in other languages, go to www.freelang.net/expressions/hello.html):

Spanish: *buenos días* or *hola*

German: *guten tag*

French: *bonjour*

Romanian: *bună ziua*

Japanese: *konnichi wa*

Italian: *ciao*

Tip: Prepare small cards with "hello" in the various native languages represented in your program. Post the cards in a place that is accessible to all for quick learning and review. Note that in many languages, there are often variations among good day, good afternoon, and good night or variations between formal and informal greetings.

The 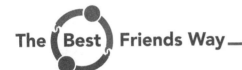 Best Friends Way _____

Life Story: When recording the life story, ask whether the *person* would enjoy a familiar greeting in his or her native language. This question can lead to other traditions of the *person,* such as whether the *person* likes to have a hug or a handshake and whether men and women greet each other in different ways.

The Arts: Make a colorful poster of written greetings in different languages.

Humor: Think of all the ways we greet each other in English, and laugh about saying "hi," "hey," or "aloha."

Sensory: Hearing familiar greetings can be stimulating.

Early Dementia: *Persons* can teach others how to say and write a particular greeting.

Conversation: Ask for advice: "Carla, am I saying 'bonjour' correctly?" Compliment: "Gerhard, I appreciate your help. I have always wanted to know how to say 'hello' in German." Laugh together: "I wonder how animals say hello?" Ask for help: "Dorothy, you speak French so well. I have a new phrase book. Would you help me learn some words?"

CHAPTER THREE

Honoring the Life Story

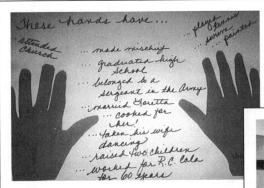

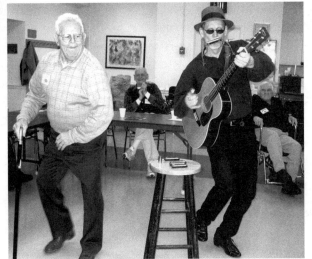

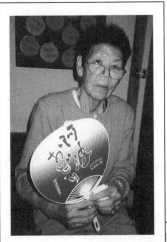

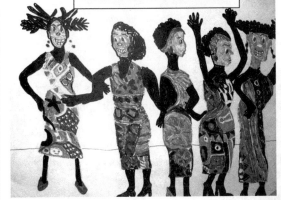

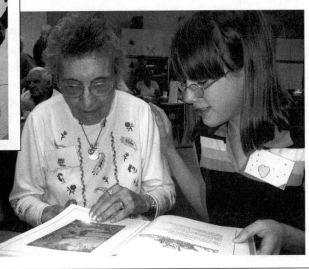

Honoring the Life Story

Friends know a lot about each other, and in a Best Friends dementia program, staff work to know well each *person* with dementia in their care. Trust and communication are enhanced when staff members know and understand each *person's* personality, family history, values and traditions, job(s), hobbies and interests, political views, spiritual beliefs, and much more.

As we have said already in the book, when *persons* feel safe, secure, and valued, and when they feel "known," challenging behaviors diminish and cooperation and community build.

Here is a quick example of the power of the life story. Contrast the two approaches:

(In a program in which staff members are not familiar with the life stories)

Staff Member: Good morning, Joe. My name is Mark. Let me help you get up and get dressed.

Joe: No. I don't need any help.

(In a program where staff members are familiar with the life stories)

Staff Member: Good morning, Joe. It's your friend Mark. I brought you your morning coffee with two sugars, just the way you like it. Hey, your favorite baseball team, the New York Yankees, won last night!

Joe: You like the Yankees, too?

Staff Member: My favorite team. Let me help you get up and get dressed today.

Joe: Sure thing!

In the second example, the staff member knew and used just a few simple facts from Joe's life story. Joe felt appreciated in that his morning drink was brought to him "just the way he liked it" and he felt known. Because this established trust, getting Joe dressed for the day goes well.

The activities in this chapter serve a dual purpose: They allow your program staff to take what they already know about *persons* in their care and put it to work. They also serve as a tool to collect new information about *persons*.

We draw your attention to a few specific activities in this chapter:

The first three activities, Things I Like (p. 36), What We Have in Common (p. 35), and Life Is a Collage (p. 38), are good ones if you are just starting to build your activity program. They are simple and fun and provide great opportunities for family involvement and information gathering about life stories.

My Old Kentucky Home (p. 41) is a good model to use to celebrate any home town or home state of a *person* in your program.

Photo Shoot (p. 50) can be a fun way to involve younger staff who may be experts at digital camera use!

Sweetheart Boulevard (p. 49) will add warmth and interest to your program space.

We believe that one of the best places to start building a better activity program is through life story work. Have fun getting to know the persons in your care—and each other!

Tips for staff training: To teach these activities, we recommend doing some as a group at staff meetings or inservice training sessions. Things I Like (p. 36), Did You Ever? (p. 40), and Photo Shoot (p. 50) are particularly successful in these environments. When staff members enjoy learning more about each other, it reinforces the benefits of learning more about *persons* who are in their care.

You can also take a resident or *person* in your program and brainstorm as many facts as you can about him or her, then discuss one interesting fact at length. For example, if you know Tap Steven, the poet mentioned in Chapter 1, then you could brainstorm how to honor his interest in poetry.

- Ask him to read one of his poems.
- Ask him to elaborate on the meaning.
- Compliment him for being the author.
- Pass around his poem or book for everyone to admire.
- Ask him where he gets his ideas.

This could lead to a number of additional activities, including composing a group poem (see Volume One, Writing Poetry, p. 51), reading famous poems, having fun with a rhyming dictionary, or talking about famous poets (e.g., many people of Scottish heritage view the poet Robert Burns as part of their heritage).

CHAPTER THREE ACTIVITIES

The Basics

- Flipchart
- Markers

Brainstorm traits and abilities that *persons* hold in common, such as birthdays, places of birth, names, foods, vacation spots, careers, places of worship, colors, sports, love of chocolate, hobbies, and colleges.

There are the obvious things that *persons* have in common, such as two women with the name of Dorothy, but there are many other ways that they have common traits, such as two *persons* who love sweets or two *persons* who knew each other in elementary school. Record on the flipchart all of the commonalities that come to mind, such as the three group members who were born in Alabama or the two who are electrical engineers.

Variation: If the group is seated at tables, have each table think of at least three things that the members of their table have in common, such as all are wearing pants, all have beautiful smiles, and everyone likes ice cream.

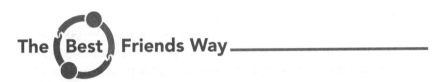

The Best Friends Way

Life Story: This is a good way for *persons* to get recognition when other strengths and abilities are slipping away. It is also a good way for the staff to learn little things about *persons* that may make much difference in their self-esteem. These common bonds can be used over and over throughout the day as *persons* are greeted or introduced to others.

The Arts: Make posters of the "twins" who both were born in Germany, the two who played football in college, and other twin combinations.

Music: Are there two people who play the same instrument or like Elvis Presley or The Beatles?

Humor: Try to think of all the ways in which *persons* have common bonds that are humorous, such as those who like to play pranks on others.

Old Sayings: "It's a small world after all!"

Old Skills: Draw attention to the common skills of *persons*, such as those who enjoy hiking or those who were schoolteachers.

Spirituality: Have *persons* been members of the same faith community or supported a common charity?

Late Dementia: This is a good way to bring everyone into the circle of positive affirmation.

Conversation: Compare: "Hiroshe, isn't it interesting that we both love to go to Florida for our vacations?" Share a secret: "I'll bet you do not know that Emily and I are members of the same church." Surprise, surprise: "Jonas and I both like to go to horse races and bet on the ponies."

What We Have in Common

Recognizing the traits that we hold in common creates a bond between us. *Persons* with dementia thrive on the recognition of common bonds among those who form their community.

Things I Like

Most of us enjoy thinking about or describing the things that we like. This is a simple exercise in handwriting whereby *persons* with dementia name the things that they like and then turn it into a handsome piece of art that they can proudly display.

The Basics

- Paper and pen to make a list
- 12" × 12" cardstock in beige (or any light color)
- 12" × 12" cardstock in black (or any dark color)
- Black pen
- Scrap of black paper (for title)
- Scrap of white paper (for title)
- Scissors
- White glue

The instructions are general guidelines and may be changed and adapted to include new ideas. To make the title heading block, cut out a square or rectangle approximately 3" × 3" or 3" × 5". Cut out the black scrap slightly larger to frame it (4" × 4" or 3.5" × 5.5"). Do the lettering "Things I Like" on the white scrap. Make the lettering fancy or decorated with dots or shadows. Attach to the black frame with white glue.

Trim ¼" away from the sides of the beige cardstock. Mount with glue to the black cardstock, centered. Glue the framed title block to the cardstock, centered, or off-center if you like.

On a separate piece of paper, make a list of things that the *person* likes. Include a variety of ideas. This list can include things all in one category, such as favorite desserts, or a list of things in general. You may list foods, colors, feelings, people, clothes, places, activities, or numbers. Anything goes. Using the black pen, write the "things" down in different sizes, different handwriting, some fancy, some plain, any way you wish around the title.

Tips: Use all acid-free materials to make a keepsake that will last for future generations. The measuring and cutting all can be done ahead of time with the help of the planning group (see Planning Group, p. 163). Use the activity informally any time a *person* needs a little personal attention.

Variations: This activity may be done as a collage using pictures or text from magazines.

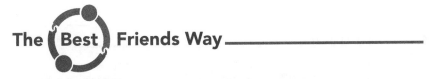
Life Story: Title the list for the *person* on the basis of something you already know about him or her. For instance, for a *person* who has been a gardener, title the list "Penelope's Perennial Flowers."

The Arts: Hang the finished product on the wall for all to see.

Music: List favorite songs, types of dances, instruments, opera, etc. Sing, "These are a few of my favorite things," from *The Sound of Music.*

Humor: Celebrate the comedian or jokester by highlighting his or her funny attributes.

Old Skills: Handwriting.

Late Dementia: *Persons* in late dementia may be able to list things that they like or may recognize words that describe things that they like.

Conversation: Share a memory: "I like sitting on the beach by the ocean in my bathing suit and feeling the warm sun and the cool breeze! Do you?" Encourage conversation: "Heber, you took so many cruises with your wife, Elayne. Let's list the countries you visited." Share something in common: "Coach, let's make a list of our favorite sports."

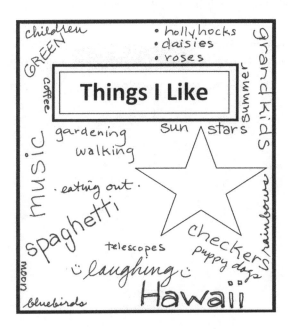

Life Is a Collage

Many of us enjoy looking at old scrapbooks, yearbooks, or pictures from the past. A life collage is created in this activity to encourage *persons* with dementia who are losing short-term memories to reminisce and discuss past and present interests. It can be a celebration of life.

The Basics

- 8½" × 11" or 12" × 12" picture of the *person* (whose life is being made into a collage)
- Miscellaneous snapshots of the *person* (if using old family photos, make photocopies or scans to preserve the originals)
- Large poster board
- Colored paper in the *person's* favorite colors
- Lists of "favorites" (see List Making, p. 22) of the *person* (e.g., foods, places, people, animals, activities, songs)
- Glue sticks
- Ribbons, stickers, buttons, greeting cards, or other nearly flat embellishments
- Pens

The project can be made one-to-one or as a small group. Lay out poster board for the background. Lay the largest picture of the *person* in the center, matting with contrasting paper if desired. Organize pictures and lists around the central picture in a pleasing manner. It is visually stimulating to overlap a few corners of the photos. Glue the pictures down on the poster board as laid out. Write captions around each picture. Use ribbons, stickers, or other items to add visual interest and to decorate and embellish the pages.

Tip: Use all acid-free materials to serve as a family historical document for the next generations. Enlarge photos ahead of time with the planning group (see Planning Group, p. 163).

Variation: Record a life story in the *person's* voice (write it first, and have the *person* read it) as a keepsake for family members.

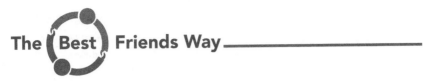

Life Story: Mine the life story for information on the *person's* interests, skills, and experiences to highlight in the collage. This project will serve as a visual life story and may be used as a tool to teach family or paid caregivers about a *person's* life.

Music: List favorite songs or types of music.

Humor: Celebrate a *person's* sense of humor by using silly pictures and telling funny stories.

Old Sayings: Does the *person* have a favorite old saying (e.g., "You bet"; "Don't bet money on that")?

Sensory: Pay attention to design details, such as making a focal point or using a color scheme, so that it will be more appealing to look at.

Spirituality: Part of being who we are is acknowledging and celebrating our heritage.

Early Dementia: Create a timeline of dates and places where the *person* lived.

Late Dementia: A *person* in late stage may be able to recognize information about his or her life and will enjoy the celebration that a life collage can provide.

Conversation: Highlight accomplishments: "Vivian, I see that you have developed many talents and skills in your life so far!" Ask for information: "Jerome, who taught you how to fish?" Compliment: "Jay, I think it is wonderful that you are so involved in Habitat for Humanity."

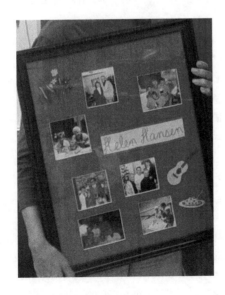

An ounce of prevention . . .

Be prepared if sad memories come up. When this happens, acknowledge the feeling and then redirect to a more positive thought.

Did You Ever?

We like to talk about our adventures. *Persons* with dementia may have trouble initiating conversation, but if a familiar event is mentioned, then they may be cued to share their stories.

The Basics

- Pen
- Slips of paper
- Fun hat

Prepare a list of "Did You Ever?" questions. Examples include ride a motorcycle, climb a mountain, ride a camel, go skinny dipping, hitchhike, chew bubble gum, play ice hockey, own a red car, or build a snow man. Put the questions in a hat.

Persons can take turns drawing a question, and, if appropriate, they can be asked to read the question. Allow plenty of time for the *person* to answer and discuss. Give everyone who wishes the opportunity to comment on the question after the *person* has finished. Because there are no right or wrong answers, everyone can feel comfortable. This also fosters reminiscing. This activity is good for a one-to-one or a small-group interaction.

Variation: The leader can ask the questions and provide an opportunity to direct some leading questions to *persons* about the stories that are known to be cherished and can be recalled if the right clues are given.

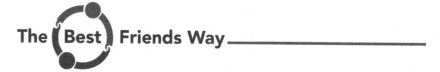

The (Best) Friends Way

Life Story: Life stories can be mined for the answer to the question "Did you ever?" Try to find as many questions as possible that can be answered with a "yes." You can also use the life story to compose "leading questions" to cue a *person,* such as, "Ray, I recall that you enjoyed hiking. Did you ever walk parts of the Appalachian trail?"

Music: Relate some questions to music, such as, "Did you ever sing in the shower?" or "Did you ever sing a solo?"

Humor: Laugh about going skinny dipping or throwing paper airplanes in class. Design some questions to be humorous.

Old Skills: Search for unique old skills to form questions, such as winning a bubble gum blowing contest.

Early Dementia: Encourage *persons* to share unique things that they have done and that are not in the hat.

Late Dementia: *Persons* may surprise you by responding to a question that is virtually failure-free.

Conversation: Provoke some discussion: "George, did you ever ride in a two-seated plane?" Reminisce: "Claudette, did you ever have to stay after school because you did not do your homework?" Ask a travel question: "Manuel, did you ever travel to Paris, France?" Encourage conversation: "Beth, did you ever eat oysters in New Orleans?" Joke in a light-hearted way: "Amanda, did you ever wish that you could win a million dollars?"

The Basics ───────────────

To prepare, research information about the state of Kentucky: state bird (cardinal), state flower (goldenrod), state capital (Frankfort), famous Kentuckians (Rosemary Clooney and Jefferson Davis), and crafts (pottery, weavers). Gather items that reflect Kentucky, such as pictures of horses, a julep cup, a Kentucky flag, and a pot of bluegrass. Prepare a traditional Kentucky food, such as derby pie, burgoo, or a hot brown.

Pass around the items and discuss each one. Highlight those in your group who were born in Kentucky. Discuss information about Kentucky and share a few fun facts, such as Cumberland Falls is the only waterfall in the Western Hemisphere to display a moonbow (a rainbow that occurs at night). Using a map, highlight each *person's* home town. Taste and discuss the traditional food. Play bluegrass music and discuss the roots of the music in Kentucky. At the close of the group, sing the state song, "My Old Kentucky Home."

Variation: The same program can be done for any location.

My Old Kentucky Home

Celebrating the history and culture of a U.S. state can teach us all about history, folklore, and regional traditions. This activity uses Kentucky as an example of a way to help the *person* with dementia celebrate his or her home state.

The (Best) Friends Way ─────────────

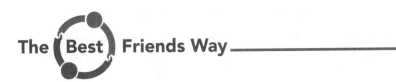

Life Story: Where in Kentucky has the *person* lived? How is his or her home town different from other parts of Kentucky? Does the *person* feel a particular connection to his or her home town through his or her family or community? Was the *person* raised in a city or a rural environment?

The Arts: Cut a poster board into the shape of the state and create a collage of Kentucky trivia or write a poem about the state on it.

Music: "Blue Moon of Kentucky," "Kentucky Rain," "Kentucky Woman," "My Old Kentucky Home."

Exercise: Identify a Kentucky landmark or state park, and visit it for a walk.

Humor: Laugh together about the fun fact that the great horse Man o' War won all of his races except one, which he lost to a horse named Upset.

Old Sayings: "Kentucky hillbilly." "Kentucky Fried Chicken."

Old Skills: Looking at a map is an old skill.

Sensory: Celebrate the bright yellow of the goldenrod and the rich taste of the Kentucky hot brown (a specialty sandwich).

Spirituality: Remembering and celebrating a *person's* roots help him or her to feel connected.

Conversation: Share information: "Marjorie, did you know that the first cheeseburger was served in Louisville?" Reminisce: "Tell me about your family vacations to Mammoth Cave." Compliment: "You must be so proud to have the county named after your great-grandfather."

Thumbprints

We all are aware of the uniqueness of our fingerprints. *Persons* with dementia respond to being special, and this activity reinforces that every *person* is "one of a kind."

The Basics

- Ink pad
- 5" × 7" cards
- Pens

Before the activity, research finger- and thumbprints. This could include when fingerprints were first used for identity, how they are read, and how they are used today. Enlarge one finger- or thumbprint to show all of the many lines that define an individual print.

Search life stories for a one- or two-word description that makes each *person* unique, such as being a master welder, having run a marathon, making coconut pancakes, having beautiful green eyes, or having a special touch with animals. Be ready to use these descriptions. Prepare cards before the activity by typing or writing this across the top: "Beverly is a unique *person* because she. . . ."

Have each *person* press his or her thumb into the ink pad and record the print in the middle of his or her 5" × 7" card. Talk about what makes each *person* so unlike anyone else and write it around the thumbprint.

Tip: Ink is available that rubs off with friction after the print is made.

Variation: Use the *person's* signature instead of the thumbprint.

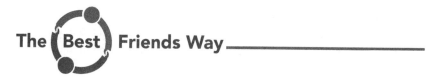

The (Best) Friends Way

Life Story: This is a wonderful opportunity to highlight special characteristics and abilities of each *person*. This card can be added to the *person's* life storybook later.

Humor: Laugh about trying to make toe prints.

Old Skills: Ask *persons* to sign their name to their creative work. Many *persons*, when asked, can sign their name and can do so beautifully.

Sensory: Make "thumbprint" cookies (typically circular cookies made from rolled dough with a center filled with jam).

Early Dementia: *Persons* can help research the facts of finger- and thumbprinting and later read aloud these facts to the group.

Conversation: Wonder together: "Vernon, do you really think that every *person* in the world has a different fingerprint?" Have fun: "Clarice, have you heard that hospitals now take footprints of newborn babies for identification? What do you think about that?" Examine: "Hobart, our fingerprints look just the same. Maybe we are related." Seek information: "Jeremy, do our fingerprints stay the same all through life?"

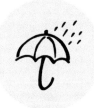

An ounce of prevention . . .

Use this activity to talk about each person's uniqueness and not to use thumbprints to decorate in a childish way.

The Basics _____

Buy a copy of *USA Today*, available at almost any newsstand. Bring it to a group environment or for a one-to-one activity. Highlight more upbeat news, the colorful weather map on the back page of section 1, the expanded sports and business sections, full-page advertisements for new cars, and local news from all 50 states and Puerto Rico.

Tie the activity to the life stories of the group. Use the weather map to chart home towns. Use the business and sports pages as activities for men who have had interest in those subjects (perhaps one is a Notre Dame graduate; look at his team's football results). Enjoy fashion ads with *persons* who like to dress well. Point out foreign news from countries where individuals grew up. Discuss commodity prices with a farmer. The possibilities are endless.

Variation: You can also discuss fun facts or trivia that often appear (e.g., 50% of all Christmas presents get returned).

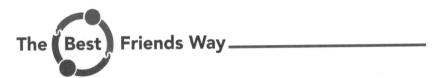

The (Best) Friends Way _____

Life Story: Who in the group regularly reads (or has read) a daily newspaper? Find out whether anyone came from a town with more than one newspaper (e.g., Chicago, New York). Does anyone enjoy crossword puzzles? Who likes to study or read the classified advertisements or advertisements for new cars? Did anyone deliver newspapers as a child?

The Arts: Use the newspaper to create a fun paper hat or paper plane. Cut up many of the colorful graphics to do a collage around sports, travel, business, or other themes (see Newspaper Art, p. 132).

Humor: Joke about any funny pictures or advertisements.

Sensory: The feel of newsprint and the rustle of a newspaper while you hold it can be pleasing. Think about the aroma of a strong morning cup of coffee while you read your morning paper.

Early Dementia: Have extended conversations about topics of the day. Read a provocative editorial together. Write a letter to the editor.

Late Dementia: Many *persons* enjoy holding a paper in their hands and turning the pages, evoking an old daily ritual.

Conversation: Compliment: "Marty, you are so smart. You stay so current with all the news." Reminisce: "Susan, look at the prices of today's cars. What did you pay for your first car?" Note commonalities: "John, let's look at the weather map in Seattle. You and I are both from that rainy city!" Share dreams: "Mr. Thompson, doesn't the Bahamas sound good right now? Let's study this advertisement and dream a bit about going to a warm beach!"

USA Today

This national newspaper has gradually gained respect and loyal readers thanks to its combination of short, catchy news items and excellent full-color graphics. *Persons* with dementia will enjoy the newspaper as a creative source of news and information to discuss and as a way to reconnect to their past lives and present interests.

Picture Memories

Enjoying pictures is a favorite pastime of many to reminisce about good times as well as pass down information about the past to the future generations. *Persons* with dementia may enjoy working with staff or family members to put together a photo album of their own.

The Basics

- Picture album
- Page protectors to fit the album
- Pictures
- Pens
- Embellishments (e.g., stickers, die-cuts)
- Glue

First, think about the type of album you would like to make. A chronological album would start with the oldest pictures first, and gradually work toward the present time. A theme album would group the pictures by themes. Pictures may also be arranged like a family tree, beginning with the first generation of photos, followed by each of the children and their families on separate pages.

Organize pictures according to the order in which they will be presented. Lay out three or four for each page. Use adhesive to adhere the pictures to the scrapbook page. Label each picture with a pen. Write actual or estimated dates on each page. Write full names of each *person* in the photos, if possible. Places and any other details about the pictures should be written down. Be creative, but set a goal that a stranger would be able to look at the book and understand the story. Add stickers or embellishments.

Don't rush the project. Take time to enjoy conversation. This activity can stretch across several shifts or several days. The activity also lends itself to volunteerism. Invite volunteers to work one-on-one with *persons* to complete this task.

Tip: Use acid-free materials so that the scrapbooks will last for many years to come.

Variations: Create postcard albums or birthday card albums using the same techniques.

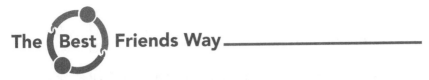
Life Story: Incorporate the stories that a *person* tells you when he or she looks at the pictures. Incorporate the *person's* favorite colors and other interests into the design of the book to personalize it. Obtain old scrapbooks from families and use them to reminisce and celebrate a *person's* past.

Humor: Include silly and funny pictures throughout the album or all on one page.

Old Sayings: "A picture is worth a thousand words."

Sensory: Looking at the pictures stimulates the senses.

Spirituality: A connection to a *person's* heritage is a spiritual connection that provides a sense of belonging.

Early Dementia: A *person* in early dementia may need help staying oriented to the sequencing of the tasks. This is a wonderful way to capture memories that are still intact.

Late Dementia: A *person* will enjoy sitting with someone and being encouraged to tell the stories to go with the pictures if he or she does not recognize the pictures. He or she may enjoy just listening to the stories told by someone else.

Conversation: Laugh together: "Jesu, look at this mustache; it really does look like a handlebar!" Ask for information: "What a wonderful wedding photo. Tell me how you met your wife." Ask a silly question: "Margie, you and your cousin look like identical twins. Did anyone mistake you for twins?"

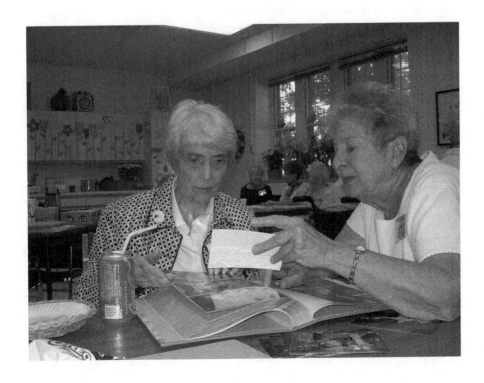

An ounce of prevention . . .

Do not ask a person to "remember" a particular event based on the pictures. Rather, ask, "What do you see happening in this picture?" Accept any answer given.

Bragging Rights

Everyone has something about which to brag. Grandchildren, an award, losing weight, or past or present accomplishments all are reasons for one to brag. *Persons* with dementia can enjoy this same sense of celebration when a friend helps them recall a "brag" story.

The Basics _____

Choose at least one brag story for each *person*. Write the story on a card for easy delivery. When appropriate, obtain a prop to support the brag story.

Call each *person* by name, and ask permission to brag about something that is very special to him or her. The brag story can be something that he or she has done or a way of life that has enhanced the lives of others. If agreeable to the *person,* then have him or her come to a central seat to be visible to everyone. After the brag story is told, the discussion can continue by asking questions: "How did you feel when you bowled a perfect 300?" or "Tell us more about your granddaughter, Mollie. I understand she makes all A's in school" or "Would you like to go back into politics?"

Tip: It is fun to ask the staff to share a brag story.

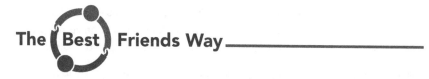

The (Best) Friends Way _____

Life Story: Mine the life story of each *person* for awards, accomplishments, values, skills, abilities, and attributes. The more familiar one becomes with each *person's* life story, the more stories emerge.

The Arts: Arrange the cards with the brag stories in an artistic way on the bulletin board for friends and families to enjoy.

Music: Brag stories can relate to many aspects of music, such as playing an instrument, directing a choir, or singing a solo.

Humor: Bragging by nature is often humorous. Maybe someone can stick out his or her tongue and touch his or her nose, or maybe someone caught that big fish that got away!

An ounce of prevention . . .

If the person does not recognize the story, then move on to another subject. Also, bringing props such as a medal or a trophy can cause the person to worry about losing the item.

Old Skills: Ask *persons* to demonstrate their skills if appropriate, such as fly fishing, playing the piano, spelling, doing crossword puzzles or "jumbles" from the newspaper, whistling, ballroom dancing, or showing off the perfect golf swing.

Spirituality: Emphasizing accomplishments can help a *person* feel that his or her life has meaning and purpose.

Conversation: Laugh together: "Now, Diane, was that fish you caught really as big as a whale?" Identify with your friend: "Delbert, you and I are just like two peas in a pod. We both have great brag stories." Ponder about a far-fetched story: "Sue, I wonder whether that story could possibly be true." Compliment: "Scott, that story was something to brag about. You deserve that medal."

The Basics _____

Collect quart-size canning jars such as mayonnaise jars or old-fashioned green canning jars. Review the life story and choose 10 to 12 favorite memories from each *person*, such as place of birth, parents' names, childhood memories, games, sports, honors, work, travel, favorite color, funny story, children, helping others, place of worship, and hobbies. Type each memory on paper that can be easily folded to fit in the jar. Pictures can also be added.

    This activity works well one-to-one or in a small group. In the group, one memory can be drawn from each *person's* jar until everyone has had a memory chosen. Read the special memory to the group and encourage discussion about it from the *person* whose memory is being highlighted, and also from others in the group. If the memory reads, "Marge met her husband on a blind date," then not only can Marge recount the whole story, but others may have opinions, suggestions, and maybe a similar experience to share.

Home-Canned Memories

Home canning of fruits and vegetables is an activity that can produce many great memories. This activity uses glass jars to hold "canned memories" of *persons* with dementia. The jars can be decorated and used individually or in a group activity to remind *persons* of happy times.

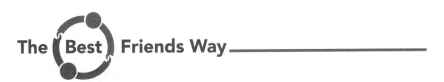

The (Best) Friends Way _____

Life Story: Did a *person* ever can fruits or vegetables or make homemade jams? Did his or her mother ever make canning a summer activity to have year-round tomatoes and other fruits and vegetables?

The Arts: As a top for the jar, cut fabric with pinking shears and tie with a colorful ribbon.

Music: When a favorite song is drawn, sing or hum to the music. If a favorite dance is drawn, then encourage the *person* to demonstrate the dance for others to enjoy and join in if they choose.

Humor: Make a joke jar full of simple, funny jokes to share.

Old Sayings: Any favorite old sayings or poems can be added to the memory jars. Recall the names of jar manufacturers, such as Ball and Mason.

Old Skills: Include stories about the skills of each *person*, such as crocheting or woodworking. Using a pressure cooker for preparing meals or sealing the jars is an old skill.

Spirituality: Add any memories of the *person's* religious experiences: baptism; singing in the church choir; the place of worship; or celebrations such as Hanukkah, Ramadan, or Christmas.

Conversation: Compliment: "Hamud, you were brave to hitch a ride on the L&N Railroad." Learn some new facts: "Grace, I never knew that the Trans-Siberian train always runs on Moscow time. You found that out the hard way." Find something in common: "Doris, I am learning that you have a twin sister, and I have a twin sister also."

An ounce of prevention . . .

Be sensitive if the memory is no longer acknowledged. Move quickly to include the person in another way.

What I Like About You

We all enjoy kind words that are given to us by friends who know us well and appreciate us for who we are. *Persons* who cannot remember many things can appreciate thoughtful expressions from others.

The Basics

Make a list ahead of time of the qualities of each *person* in your group.

Put each *person's* name in a hat. Take turns drawing a name from the hat. When appropriate, let the participant who draws the name announce the name drawn.

Draw attention to the *person* whose name is drawn, repeat his or her name, and ask the group to think of some things that they like about him or her. If there is not a quick response, then look at your own list and say "What do you think of Chuck's kind words?" or "What about Dora's love of family?" Discuss any particular stories related to the positive attributes that you know to be familiar to him or her.

The 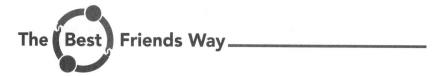 Best Friends Way

Life Story: This is a great way to bring attention to the caring, compassionate side of *persons* and mention specific values held, such as hard work, honesty, kindness, and generosity. It is an excellent way to become more familiar with each *person's* life story.

The Arts: Write "What I Like About You" in calligraphy, including each *person's* name. Mount the responses on a poster board for display.

Music: Think of all the ways in which *persons* are related to music, such as playing an instrument, listening to an opera or country music, loving to sing and dance, or marching in the high school band.

Humor: For a fun twist, name one quality that makes each *person* irresistible.

Old Skills: Any old skills, such as kayaking or playing a competitive game of checkers, make good answers to the game of "What I Like About You."

Spirituality: Low self-esteem can often accompany dementia. Hearing nice comments about oneself can lift the spirit. This may be a good time to comment on a *person's* love of his or her particular faith community and to talk about some specific work that he or she did to help others as a member of his or her church, synagogue, or mosque.

Early Dementia: Remind *persons* what their family and community like about them.

Late Dementia: Hearing their preferred name and a compliment can evoke a positive response.

Conversation: Recall a good deed: "Desmond, your support of the Hill 'n Dale swimming pool made it possible for hundreds of children to take swimming lessons and learn to swim. What a gift to the community." Take note: "Macala, I like the way you guide Paul's wheelchair. It makes him feel so safe." Note busy hands: "Rose, you are always busy helping others. You are my model."

The Basics ————————————

- Construction paper, red and pink
- Glue
- Scissors
- Photocopies of a wedding photo or the *person* with his or her significant other

If the *person* is single or divorced, then ask the *person* who his or her favorite celebrity is and feature the *person* with a picture of that celebrity. Alternatively, ask whether there is a type of "dream person" whom a *person* would want to include in the photo display with him or her. It is also great to include a favorite pet or animal. Use your imagination!

   Cut the copied photo into a heart shape and write the couple's names in or around the photo. Glue or tape onto a mat made from the red or pink construction paper. Choose a hallway or wall as your Sweetheart Boulevard. Staff members are also welcome to share their sweethearts!

Submitted by Jean L. McInnis, Activity Coordinator, Gorham House, Gorham, ME.

Sweetheart Boulevard

Almost all of us have had a sweetheart in our life—or more than one! This activity celebrates everyone's "sweethearts." Hanging wedding photos or other photos of close friends on a wall renamed "Sweetheart Boulevard" can be a year-round event or be done especially for Valentine's Day.

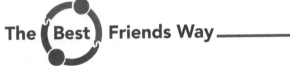

The (Best) Friends Way ————————————

Life Story: Review the *person's* life story to know of significant others in their lives that may be appropriate for the Sweetheart Boulevard. Mine the life story for information on the relationship, such as how they met or how long they have known each other.

The Arts: Create a decorative frame or mat for the pictures. Use shell-textured frames for the pictures (see Eggshell Picture Frames, p. 131).

Music: Play familiar love songs as background music as you talk about sweethearts, or sing songs such as "Let Me Call You Sweetheart" or "I Can't Help Loving You."

Exercise: Take a walk each day to visit Sweetheart Boulevard and reminisce.

Humor: Discuss first dates or blind dates. Share some funny stories about the *person's* wedding ceremony or early days of their relationship.

Old Sayings: "Love makes the world go round." "Love is blind."

Conversation: Laugh together: "Helen, I love the story of when your husband proposed to you at the Eiffel Tower!" Celebrate the relationship: "Jim, how special that you and Judy have been married for 62 years." Have fun: "Mike, I know a man's best friend is his dog. Your dog is a true sweetheart!"

An ounce of prevention . . .

If the person did not have a significant other, then work with him or her to determine who to include in a picture with him or her.

Photo Shoot

This activity is an easy way to capture a photograph of each *person*. It is fun for the *person* with dementia and entertainment for the whole group.

The Basics

- Camera (digital is best)
- Tripod (optional)
- Simple background
- Good light
- Comfortable chair
- Printer for digital camera (optional)

Arrange a "portrait studio" in a place in the room that is quiet and free from clutter and that has good light for photography. Set up a comfortable chair. Select a good place for the camera and use a tripod or other stable support so that the camera will not have to be moved as the models change. Involve the group as an audience while each *person* poses for his or her photograph. Post pictures on a bulletin board, use in a collage, and/or send pictures to families.

Variations: You can use simple props to jazz up the photos, such as a hat or a scarf. Props can add humor or formality to the portraits.

The 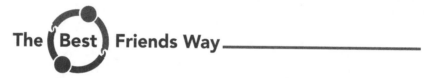 Best Friends Way

Life Story: Explore all of the reasons that a *person* may have had his or her picture taken throughout his or her life, such as church directories, driver's licenses, work name badges, school pictures, and graduation pictures. Know the photography style of the period in which the *person* grew up to spark discussion of the old ways.

Humor: Take a silly portrait together.

Old Sayings: "Smile, you're on 'Candid Camera'!" I wouldn't want you to "break the camera."

Sensory: The occasion can be quite social and invite much give and take, kidding, and good humor.

Early Dementia: The *person* may enjoy being the photographer or helping set up the background for the shot.

Late Dementia: Help a *person* look his or her best by combing hair or adding a little make-up.

Conversation: Refer to a long-term memory: "Miss Lilly, did you ever use a box camera?" Share a secret: "Did you show anyone those girly pin-ups that we used to hang inside our locker?" Ask with a smile: "George, do you carry a picture of your girlfriend in your wallet?"

An ounce of prevention . . .

The person *may not recognize him- or herself in the picture. Note that* some persons *have never wanted to have their picture taken.*

The Basics ─────────────

- Paper
- Pencils

Research facts about the hands. Topics could include the number of muscles and bones in each hand, the importance of the thumb in evolution, or the uniqueness of palm lines or fingerprints. Create tracings of different-sized hands. In the group, take a moment to look at different-sized hands and talk about how important our hands are to us. Have each *person* trace his or her hands on a sheet of paper with a pencil. Inside the hand, on the sheet of paper, or wherever they choose, write all of the things that their hands have done, for example, raised children, wrote on a chalkboard, built a crib for a grandchild, played golf, or conducted an orchestra. See a photograph of this activity in the collage at the beginning of this chapter.

Hands Up!

Our hands hold the secrets of the activities and accomplishments of our life. Exploring hands can be a wonderful way to reconnect *persons* with dementia with their past successes and accomplishments.

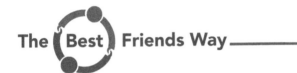

The (Best) Friends Way ─────────────

Life Story: Be familiar with *persons'* life stories to celebrate all of the things that their hands have done. Find out whether anyone earned a living as a typist or a secretary and how many words per minute they could type. Did anyone play piano or guitar? Did anyone do woodworking or needlepoint?

The Arts: Create a hand using scrap paper art (see Volume One, Scrap Paper Art, p. 58).

Exercise: Lead a finger exercise and talk about the muscles in the hand.

Humor: Laugh about what it means to be "a handful."

Old Sayings: Think of all the sayings that include the word *hand*: "Hands down," "A bird in the hand is worth two in the bush." On poster boards, put old sayings about hands and hang them around the room.

Old Skills: Practice an old skill such as quilting while reminiscing about all of the things that a *person's* hands have done.

Sensory: Give a hand massage.

Spirituality: Encourage all present to shake hands with the *person* next to them. Discuss the symbolic meaning behind the handshake.

Late Dementia: Put lotion on a *person's* hand while discussing things that he or she has enjoyed doing.

Conversation: Ask for information: "What are all of the names of each finger?" Speculate: "I wonder why a horse's height is measured in hands?" Laugh together: "Laura, what does it mean to be caught red-handed?" Compliment: "Dr. Zimmer, your hands have saved the lives of many people. You are a wonderful surgeon."

CHAPTER FOUR

Religious and Spiritual Traditions

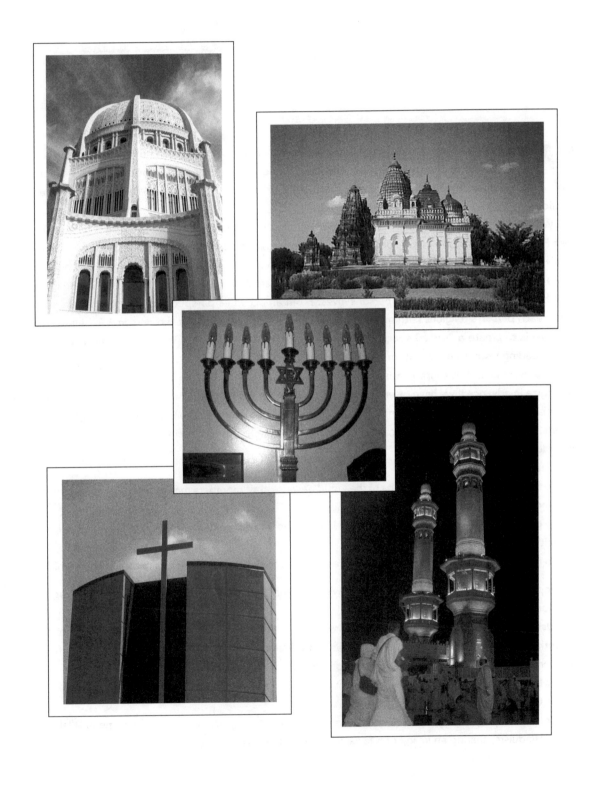

Religious and Spiritual Traditions

When reviewing books and materials on dementia care, we realized that not much has been written about spiritual and religious activities. One colleague advised us not to write this chapter because it is so challenging to summarize briefly many complex beliefs. He concluded, "Besides . . . you are bound to offend someone!"

We believe that although not everyone is part of a faith community, every one of us has a spirit. The Best Friends model of care helps *persons* fulfill their spiritual needs through art, nature, and friends and family. We have emphasized that treating each *person* with infinite value is a spiritual act in and of itself. However, many *persons* have been or are active and dedicated members of a faith community. Religious faith has been the center of many *persons'* lives. From an activities perspective, our goal should be to honor each *person's* religious faith or traditions as long as it has meaning for the *person*. We believe that our goal is to create a "sacred space," and that this can be as simple as singing a meaningful religious hymn, reading from a sacred text, or helping someone with his or her prayer beads.

The material in this chapter was written in consultation with practicing members of each faith. We apologize in advance if we have offended any sensibilities. The challenge is one of diversity. For example, Christianity has many faith communities, and within those communities there are churches with diverse beliefs. With each religion, however, we tried to find a common prayer, blessing, or ritual that transcends individual differences.

Our goals for this chapter are:

1. To introduce many of the religions of the world because staff members may increasingly serve *persons* who come from unfamiliar faith communities.
2. To give staff members one or two valuable ideas on how to connect each *person* to his or her religious faith.
3. To recognize that staff members themselves come from diverse backgrounds and faith communities.

We hope that the information in this chapter will help us all get to know one another better and respect and honor differences.

Using these activities is pretty straightforward. In The Basics for each activity, we have one or two essential points. Hopefully, these ideas are ones that will be the most familiar and the most meaningful for the *person*, even late into dementia. Examples include:

- for Buddhism, reading or discussing the Four Noble Truths
- for Christianity, praying the Lord's Prayer
- for Islam, saying the significant phrase, Bismillah (bis-MIL-lah), which means "in the name of Allah"
- for Hinduism, sharing an image of a favorite deity, such as Vishnu or Shiva

In The Best Friends Way (part of each activity), other traditions and rituals are noted. *Persons* with dementia generally respond well to ritual, be it having breakfast at a certain time of day or exercise class at 11 a.m. Similarly, long-learned and practiced religious rituals may be comforting, such as prayers or certain blessings before meals or prayer beads.

Tips for staff training: Give special attention to anyone in your program who may have a religion that is unique to the group (e.g., if your day center has only one member of the Baha'i faith). He or she would appreciate a staff member's interest in and respect of his or her traditions.

Individual activities in this chapter can be used as an orientation for staff members to raise their awareness about diverse faiths (of *persons* or of each other) or to celebrate a religious holiday. They can also be turned into classroom activities (see Chapter 6, "Adult Education," for ideas); everyone present can enjoy this version of a "comparative religion" class!

A word of caution: Discuss boundaries with staff when it comes to sharing their own beliefs. It is good to inform and connect but never appropriate to impose your beliefs on others.

CHAPTER FOUR ACTIVITIES

The Basics _____

Following are two familiar prayers/blessings of the Baha'i faith to use to connect a *person* to his or her faith:

Allah'u'Abha (ah-LA-ho AB-ha) is an Arabic phrase that means "God is most glorious." It is used among Baha'i followers as a greeting, a prayer, and a blessing. This is used by Baha'is in every country, regardless of local language.

"O God! Guide me, protect me. Make of me a shining lamp and a brilliant star. Thou are the Mighty and the Powerful." This prayer is used to ask for God's guidance and protection and is a reminder of God's blessings. It can help ease someone who is anxious or fearful. This prayer in English is often memorized by Baha'is.

The (Best) Friends Way _____

Life Story: The *person* may enjoy recalling the celebration of the Baha'i New Year (Naw Ruz, pronounced "norh ROOZ") on March 21. Did he or she go on a Baha'i Pilgrimage to Haifa and Acca in Israel, a time when individuals visit the holy shrines of the Bab and Baha'u'llah?

The Arts: Pictures of the Shrine of the Bab on Mt. Carmel in Haifa, surrounded by beautiful gardens and fountains, are treasured by *persons* of this faith.

Music: The *person* may enjoy familiar songs or chanted prayers that are made available by family members. Also recordings of Baha'i prayers sung or set to music are available commercially.

Sensory: It is common for *persons* to have prayer beads made from various materials. Holding the beads not only reminds one of his or her faith but also can be stimulating to the touch. The aroma of roses and jasmine will be sensory pleasing because these flowers are planted in and near the Holy Shrines in Israel and in the gardens that surround the Baha'i houses of worship throughout the world.

Early Dementia: *Persons* can read from the sacred writings known as The Hidden Words or help with a program on the Baha'i faith.

Late Dementia: Saying the phrases above with reverence and love would be understood and appreciated even if the *person* did not speak or outwardly respond. In the Baha'i religion, Baha'u'llah teaches that the soul has a life and a consciousness that remain unimpaired by physical limitations.

Conversation: Demonstrate your interest in the faith of another: "Luis, tell me how you became a Baha'i." Compliment: "Margaret, I know you were a tutor of Ruhi (ROO-he) books and classes. I am proud of you for giving your time to guide others in learning more about your faith." Ask for help: "Ian, Baha'is have prayers that they say each day. Can you help me with this short noonday prayer?"

Written in consultation with Marianne Smith Geula, Esq., LLM, Chicago, IL.

Baha'i Faith

Followers of the Baha'i faith believe that Baha'u'llah is the most recent in a succession of divine messengers from God. His message is one of unity, teaching that there is only one God and one human race and that all of the world's religions represent stages in the revelation of God's will. *Persons* with dementia may find reassurance from a familiar blessing or prayer.

Buddhism

Buddhism is based on the teachings of the Buddha, the Awakened One, Siddhartha Gotama. Buddhism is a path that teaches a way of life that guides one to live an awakened life through pure living and thinking based on morality, meditation, and wisdom. *Persons* with dementia may find comfort in familiar teachings of their faith and from the serenity of the Buddhist way of life.

The Basics

There are many different traditions within Buddhism, but one common thread is the teaching of the Four Noble Truths. The *person* may appreciate reading them alone or having someone read them aloud.

The Four Noble Truths:
1. There is suffering in the human condition.
2. There is reason for such suffering.
3. There is a way out of suffering.
4. The eight-fold path is the way out of suffering (being moral through what we say and do, focusing the mind on being aware of our thoughts and actions, and developing wisdom and understanding).

Persons may also appreciate hearing the Three Jewels of Buddhism:
1. I take refuge in the Buddha, the one who shows me the way in this life.
2. I take refuge in the Dharma, the way of love and understanding.
3. I take refuge in the Sangha, the community that lives in harmony and awareness.

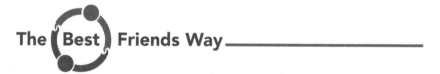

The (Best) Friends Way

Life Story: Because of the many different traditions within Buddhism, it is very important for the life story to detail the particular traditions that remain meaningful to the *person*. Was the person born into a Buddhist tradition or did he or she come to it independently?

The Arts: Ask a family member to bring some objects that are used in traditional Buddhist rituals, such as prayer flags made by Tibetan monks or thangka (Tibetan paintings of various scenes of the Buddha and his disciples).

Music: Sounding a bell or gong is traditional in Buddhism. Chant familiar phrases: "Om Mane Padme Hung" or "Gate Gate Paragate Parasamgate Bodhi Swaha."

Sensory: The aroma of incense, the feel of prayer beads, or the sounds of running water, a bell, or a gong provide sensory stimulation and may trigger memories.

Late Dementia: *Persons* may enjoy holding a statue of the Buddha, a prayer wheel, or prayer beads (known as mala beads).

Conversation: Encourage conversation: "Ramiro, have you ever met a Buddhist monk?" Share something in common: "Lee, when I was in Japan, I visited a Buddhist temple. It was very ornate. Have you visited many temples?" Explore: "Dr. Fluno, I am told you became a Buddhist at the age of 50. Tell me more about that."

Written in consultation with Corinne Rovetti, RNCS/FNP, Knoxville, TN.

The Basics ———————————

The one prayer that cuts across all expressions of the Christian faith is the prayer that Jesus taught to his disciples, commonly known as the Lord's prayer. Christians learn it at an early age. There are slight variations, so check for what is most familiar or choose another prayer if more appropriate for the *person.*

> Our Father who art in heaven, hallowed be thy name.
> Thy kingdom come. Thy will be done, on earth as it is in Heaven.
> Give us this day our daily bread. And forgive us our trespasses, as
>   we forgive them that trespass against us.
> And lead us not into temptation, but deliver us from evil.
> For Thine is the kingdom, the power, and the glory forever. Amen.

This prayer can be found in Matthew, Chapter 6, and Luke, Chapter 11. Other very familiar parts of the Bible are Psalm 23 and the 13th Chapter of I Corinthians. Read from these passages if the *person* is comforted by hearing these very familiar words.

Christianity

Christians believe in one God who created the entire world and lived among people in the person of Jesus of Nazareth. Jesus taught that God is a God of love, compassion, mercy, and forgiveness. God experiences our humanity and identifies with the good things in our life as well as our pain and suffering. *Persons* with dementia often are comforted by familiar prayers and rituals from their faith.

The 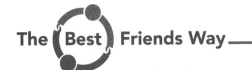 Best Friends Way ———————————

Life Story: Find out if the *person* attended church often and which denomination it was (e.g., Baptist, Methodist, Catholic). Did he or she attend a youth group or sing in a choir as a child? Does the family celebrate Easter and Christmas in a special way?

The Arts: Bring in art books or reproductions of famous artistic portrayals of the life and works of Jesus to share with the group. Bring in a collection of crosses and beautiful Catholic rosaries to enjoy and discuss.

Music: Hearing or singing familiar hymns can be a strong reminder of one's faith, even when the words may no longer have meaning.

Humor: Reminisce about the time someone fell asleep during a long sermon.

Sensory: Some traditional foods served at Christmas time, such as eggnog and plum pudding, can be a feast for the taste buds. Enjoy the lights and decorations of a Christmas tree.

Early Dementia: *Persons* can participate in a worship service by reading from the Bible. They may also appreciate helping with plans for a worship service.

Late Dementia: It may be comforting for a *person* to hold a Bible, a cross, or another religious item, such as a rosary for *persons* of the Catholic faith.

Conversation: Reminisce: "Talbott, did you attend Sunday school when you were growing up?" Share something in common: "Daisy, we are both members of the Catholic Church. Did you have Catholic nuns for teachers like I did?" Ponder together: "Cole, I wonder why some churches have tall spires."

Written in consultation with Dr. William O. Paulsell, President Emeritus, Lexington Theological Seminary, Lexington, KY.

Confucianism

Confucianism, which originated in approximately the 5th century BC, is an ancient philosophy, a set of principles to ensure ethical relationships and practices among and between individuals, families, and government. *Persons* with dementia will feel a sense of comfort and reassurance when they are connected to these principles.

The Basics

There are Five Constant Relationships that make up the fabric of the Confucian way of life: those between parent and child, husband and wife, elder sibling and junior sibling, elder friend and junior friend, and ruler and ruled. Above all other virtues of Confucianism is the virtue of *filial devotion,* a son's or daughter's respect or devotion to his or her parents. Confucius taught that all other moral virtues, indeed civilization itself, flows from filial devotion.

One way to connect a *person* with this way of life is for a caregiver to show the kind of devotion instilled in children for all older people, especially parents, including joyful attention, respect, and reverence.

Because so much emphasis in Confucianism is placed on the family, engage the *person* in conversation about his or her family. Look at family pictures, and reminisce about the family.

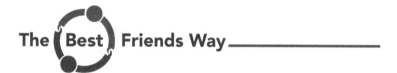

The (Best) Friends Way

Life Story: In compiling the *person's* life story, try to be specific about what in this tradition has the most meaning to the *person.* Has anyone visited a Confucian temple? Who has traveled to China, Taiwan, or nearby countries?

The Arts: Show colorful pictures of the Forbidden City, especially the beautiful circular, three-tiered Altar of Heaven in the Temple of Heaven compound in Beijing, China. Display Confucian landscape paintings and encourage everyone to paint their own version.

Music: Look at, listen to, or play one of the traditional Eight Musical Instruments, including a musical stone, a bell, a drum, a reed organ, a lute, a flute, an ocarina, and a percussion instrument.

Sensory: In Confucian tradition, a set of five colors—red, gold, white, green, and black—have special association. Ask a *person* to read a short description of the meaning of the colors and experience the vividness of each color.

Early Dementia: A *person* could share information about a Confucian temple or the Chinese lunar calendar, with its 12 animals of the Chinese zodiac.

Conversation: Encourage conversation: "Did your family attend the celebration on September 28 for Confucius's birthday when you lived in Taiwan?" Compliment: "Donna, I love the picture of you and your family taken in front of the temple in Beijing." Learn from each other: "Kim, how did your parents teach you to honor and respect all older people?"

Written in consultation with Rong-Chi Chen, MD, Professor of Neurology, National Taiwan University, and Honorary President, Taiwan Alzheimer's Disease Association, Taipei, Taiwan.

The Basics

One of the most universal rituals and one that may resonate the longest for *persons* of this faith is to give the *person* a picture or an image to hold of a favorite deity, such as Vishnu, Shiva, Durga, Krishna, Ganesha, Hanuman, or Kartikeya. It is believed that these deities, or gods, represent different expressions of Brahman, or the one God. Hearing some verses from the sacred books of Hinduism—The Bhagavad-Gita, Ramayana, and The Veda—can also be reassuring to *persons* with dementia.

Hinduism

Hindus believe in a universal soul or God called Brahman, the pure consciousness, the eternal origin who is the cause and the foundation of all existence. That existence is a cycle of birth, death, and rebirth. *Persons* with dementia may find comfort and solace in some of the traditions and rituals of their faith.

The 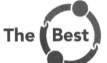 Best Friends Way

Life Story: Different Hindu communities may have their own divinities that they worship. These deities, according to Hinduism, are simply different ways of approaching the Ultimate. It is important that the life story note the particular deities worshipped by each *person* of this faith. What memories does one have of a shrine for worship in his or her home? What does the *person* remember about worshipping at a temple?

The Arts: Deities of the Hindu faith are very colorful. Collect pictures or images of some deities, and let *persons* tell about the meaning of each one. Also, Hindu temples are often very ornate with interesting architecture. Provide a picture of a temple for all to enjoy.

Music: Listening to religious songs, called bhajan, is a way of remembering/praying to gods and may be very soothing.

Sensory: *Persons* of the Hindu faith often say aloud the names of their favorite gods and repeat mantras—sacred sayings repeated in prayer or meditation. The sounds of mantras repeated over and over can be consoling and are believed to be purifying for the soul.

Early Dementia: *Persons* can help lead a discussion on many aspects of the faith, such as explaining the meaning of *karma* (proper ritual and ethical actions as a means to spiritual progress).

Conversation: Share together: "Geeta, here is a picture of Gandhi. He was a devout Hindu and did so much good for many people." Ask for information: "Ram, did you have a certain time of day to worship at the shrine in your home?" Ponder: "Hinduism is such an old religion. I wonder how it was handed down without the written word." Ask for information: "Manoj, did your family wear the 'sacred thread' when they worshipped?" (Some Hindus do, some do not.)

Written in consultation with Vinod Srivastava, Family Services, Providence, RI.

An ounce of prevention . . .

Persons of the Hindu faith often are vegetarian and do not eat beef because of a religious belief. Take precautions to honor these traditions.

Islam

Muslims believe in one God and that the prophet Mohammad is his last and final messenger. *Persons* with dementia who are of the religion known as Islam may find reassurance from a familiar saying, prayer, or ritual of their faith.

The Basics

Following are two short phrases that help connect *persons* to this faith. They should be said in Arabic, noting the pronunciation guide in parentheses.

Al-hamdulillah (al-ham-DU-lil-lah) means "Praise Allah." Muslims typically say this whenever they think of, speak of, or hear something good, to remind themselves that everything good comes from Allah.

Bismillah (bis-MIL-lah) means "In the name of Allah." Muslims often say this before eating, drinking, or embarking on any significant activity.

The 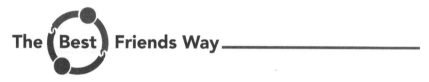 Best Friends Way

Life Story: Try to learn from the family the special memories that the *person* has retained of the practice of his or her faith. The *person* may enjoy recalling Ramadan, a time when Muslims fast during the daytime for a month and focus on their spirituality. Did he or she make a pilgrimage to Mecca (hajj) to visit the holy Ka'ba, the mosque built by Abraham?

The Arts: Pictures of the Ka'ba, surrounded by worshippers, can be a delight for *persons* to see and discuss.

Music: The call to prayer is a rhythmic sound that is familiar to every Muslim of any culture. Ask a family member to provide a recording of the call to prayer.

Sensory: A misbaha (prayer beads) is often used by Muslims to give thanks to Allah, to ask for forgiveness, or simply to glorify him through phrases that are uttered while counting the beads. A *person* may enjoy reading from the Quran (Koran) written in Arabic.

Early Dementia: A *person* may enjoy telling the group about a trip to Mecca or showing others the characters in the Arabic language.

Late Dementia: The tone and cadence of the blessings, prayers, and recitation of the Quran will have meaning even if the words no longer seem to be understood.

Conversation: Reminisce: "Fatima, tell me about fasting during the month of Ramadan. Did you look forward to the evening meal after fasting all day?" Ask for help: "Mohammad, can you help me spell Ramadan for this announcement?" Ponder together: "I wonder why a mosque has a dome and a church has a spire." Ask for help: "Amira, I do not know how to read in Arabic. Would you read this passage from the Quran for me?"

Written in consultation with Samieh Shalash, reporter, The Winchester Sun, Winchester, KY.

An ounce of prevention . . .

The prayers and blessings need to be said in Arabic and will be appreciated even if one struggles with pronunciation. Persons will probably be able, once you initiate a saying, to help you with the Arabic.

The Basics _____

The Sh'ma is recited traditionally during the morning and evening prayer service, as one goes to sleep at night, and even on the deathbed. It is one of the first Jewish prayers that young children learn.

> SH'MA YISRA-EL ADONAI ELO-HAY-NU ADONAI ECHAD
> Hear, O Israel, Adonai is our God, Adonai is One

The following blessing is used in celebration of a special birthday, anniversary, or moment of life:

> BA-RUKH ATA ADONAI ELO-HAY-NU MELEKH HA-OLAM SHEH-HEH-KHE-YANU V'KEE-Y'MANU V'HEE-GEE-ANU LAZ'-MAN HA-ZEH
> Praised are You Adonai, our God, Ruler of the Universe, for granting us the gift of life, for sustaining us, and for helping us to reach this day.

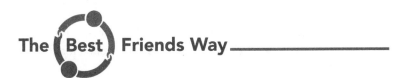

The (Best) Friends Way _____

Life Story: Was the *person's* family observant (e.g., keeping kosher, going to temple)? Did the *person* grow up in a family that celebrated Shabbat together? Did they light the candles and say Kiddush over wine? Who has a fond memory of celebrating Passover by having a special meal together? Who has visited Israel?

The Arts: Enjoy the design and meaning of the Kipa or Yarmulka (head covering) and the beauty of the Talit, a prayer shawl that is worn during prayer, especially during the Sabbath worship. Make a Star of David.

Music: Enjoy a traditional game and song for Hanukkah involving a small top with Hebrew letters on each side, called a *dreidel*.

Sensory: Taste honey-dipped apples, eaten on Rosh ha-Shana (Jewish New Year) for a sweet new year, and the Challa, a braided golden egg bread eaten on the Sabbath and other holidays. Hear the Shofar, a ram's horn blown on Rosh ha-Shana.

Early Dementia: Invite a *person* to read brief descriptions, prepared ahead of time, about the meaning of Shabbat, a "Chai," a Tzedaka Box, a Menora, Passover, or other selected material.

Late Dementia: Even though the words may have lost the meaning, the rhythm and resonance of the very familiar Jewish blessings will be felt.

Conversation: Reminisce: "Mr. Rosenberg, did you have a Bar Mitzvah when you were young?" Help me understand: "Julia, what does it mean to 'keep kosher'?" Encourage conversation: "Larry, do you have your own Talit?"

Written in consultation with Rabbi Sharon Cohen, Ohavay Zion Synagogue, Lexington, KY.

Judaism

Fundamental to Judaism is a belief in a personal connection to God. Judaism teaches that all of us are created in the image of God and have the responsibility to treat one another with dignity and respect. Judaism also teaches that humans are partners with God in the process of Creation, and we have both the responsibility and the gift of helping to make the world a better place. *Persons* with dementia will find peace and comfort in the following selections.

Native American Spirituality

Native Americans' beliefs and practices form an integral and seamless part of their very being. To them, all of life is sacred. Every living thing—the Earth and all of its inhabitants—is spirit filled. *Persons* with dementia may feel a spiritual connection when others talk with them about their beliefs.

The Basics

Native American spirituality involves respect for the wisdom of elders, the concept of family responsibility extending beyond the nuclear family to embrace the whole village, respect for the environment, and the willingness to share what they have with others. Talk with *persons* about these values.

A *person* of the Native American tradition may appreciate hearing or saying this prayer:

O' Great Spirit,
Whose voice I hear in the winds,
And whose breath gives life to all the world.
Hear me!
I am small and weak.
I need your strength and wisdom.

(This prayer is from the Red Cloud Native Americans and was published with permission in Virginia Bell's and David Troxel's article, "Spirituality and the *Person* with Dementia," *Alzheimer's Care Quarterly*/Spring 2001.)

Variation: Many of the spiritual ideas from Native Americans have links to or resonance with indigenous peoples from around the world.

The 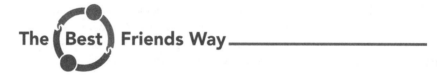 Best Friends Way

Life Story: Native Americans live in various locations with often very different traditions and rituals even though their value systems tend to remain the same. Which particular rituals are familiar to *persons* in your group who are Native American? Does the *person* know any Native American music or poetry or speak a language, such as Navajo?

The Arts: Enjoy pictures of traditional Native American pottery, baskets, or rugs. Study the many intricate designs and try to replicate some of them. Collect pictures of various Native American ceremonial dress and headwear.

Music: Talk about the drum and its part in Native American rituals. Let each *person* try beating a drum.

Sensory: Go outside and listen to the sounds and songs of nature. Comment on the whistling of the wind, the clap of the thunder, and the song of the bird.

Conversation: Ask for information: "Birdie, why do you refer to the Earth as Mother Earth?" Compliment: "Malcolm, you hear sounds of nature that I have always overlooked. You are teaching me so much. Thank you." Reminisce: "Minnie, tell me about the reservation in South Dakota where you grew up. Did you ever take part in a traditional drum corps?"

Written in consultation with Minnie Jim, Native American Outreach Coordinator, Sun City, AZ.

CHAPTER FIVE

Wellness

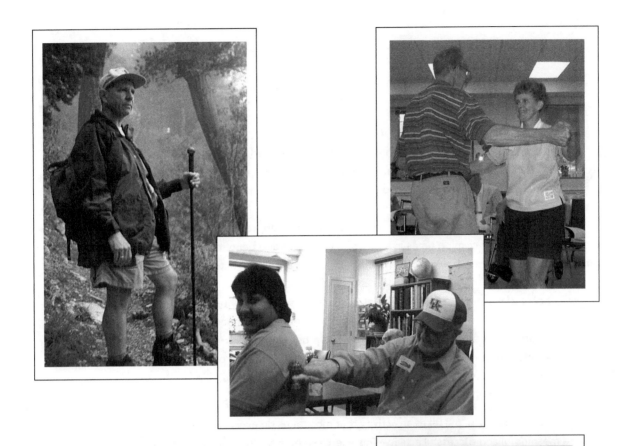

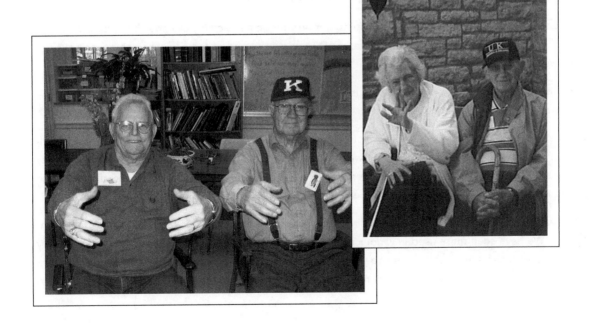

Wellness

Massages, exercise, deep breathing, the scent of a flavored candle, laughter—all of these bring quality to our life and help us feel better, particularly when we are under stress. *Persons* with dementia also benefit from pampering and wellness activities that are associated with a spa or relaxing vacation.

The wellness activities in this chapter may also benefit sleep, reduce challenging behaviors, and in general evoke quiet and calming times in a *person's* life. An added benefit of these activities is that staff members who participate will also receive the benefits. These wellness activities may help everyone stop and smell the roses and shake off some of the stress of their daily lives.

The concept of wellness may not immediately make sense in the context of Alzheimer's disease. The activities in this chapter will not stop the progression of dementia, but many believe that wellness activities such as these do no harm, fight depression, and help *persons* function at their very best. These activities, such as intentional walking, also build physical strength, may help prevent falls, and lower excess disability. For younger *persons*, these activities may already be part of their life.

We draw your attention to a few specific activities in this chapter:

Daily Intentional Walking (p. 69) takes an activity that most of us do every day and describes how to make it a more meaningful and successful activity. This exercise benefits all involved and can be an opportunity for volunteer recruitment because many retirees enjoy a daily walk.

Relaxation Hour (p. 70) is an excellent activity to put on your posted activity calendar, because that makes it part of your daily or weekly routine. It works well toward the end of the day, when some *persons* get restless.

We like A Day at the Spa (p. 72) because it is festive and something to which many in the group, particularly women, will relate.

Aromatherapy has become a cottage industry, with books, Web sites, and oils and candles widely available. The benefits may be overstated, but we think that the sensory stimulations (perhaps at the heart of many ancient principles of herbal medicines and relaxation) have healing properties and discuss these ideas in an activity called Stop and Smell the Roses (p. 76).

The reader will also note some Asian-inspired activities such as Tai Chi (p. 82) and Guided Relaxation (p. 80). We have seen these used in various environments with great success. Of note is that community practitioners may be available to come to your program to lead a Tai Chi class or wellness activity. Be sure that they have received a basic orientation on dementia so that they know how best to relate to the *per-*

sons in the activity (e.g., go slowly, keep instructions simple). Also, check with your local adult education program; it may be able to offer a class on wellness in your environment, benefiting all who participate.

Harry Nelson, who has early dementia and is featured in Chapter 1, thrives on being out-of-doors in nature, hiking, and camping. Although his cognitive ability is changing, his body remains strong. Keeping someone such as Harry socially engaged and involved in movement, music, laughter, or other wellness activities is the goal of quality care.

How you present these activities is a key factor in their success. Many *persons* with dementia are of an age or from a time when massages and spa experiences were not common. Indeed, many Depression-era elders might resist something seen as self-indulgent. Present the activities in a wellness mode or incorporate some ideas around fitness or rehabilitation. See some of the Conversation sections for more ideas on how to encourage participation in activities that may be new to some.

Tips for staff training: Many of the activities in this chapter lend themselves to a short, 15-minute session at a staff meeting; do them both to model the activity and to give staff a lift. Your agency or company may also want to develop a staff wellness program to accompany this theme (e.g., around weight loss, eating right, and other healthful lifestyle choices).

CHAPTER FIVE ACTIVITIES

The Basics _____

Create a walking club of individuals who are able and interested in participating in daily walks. Give the club a name, such as the Sacramento Striders or Miami Milers. Decide together where you will walk and when each day you will do it. Be creative in planning daily walks, such as exploring a gentle path around a park's lake or walking the halls of a local shopping mall off hours. Create a map or list to check off all of the places the club has walked. Keep a log book that the person can sign (or check off his or her name) each day showing the total miles he or she has walked to foster a sense of accomplishment.

Variations: Consider creating a men's walking club for an activity that encourages their involvement.

Daily Intentional Walking

Setting aside time to exercise each day is good for all of us. *Persons* with dementia, who cannot always initiate the activity, benefit from a daily intentional walk.

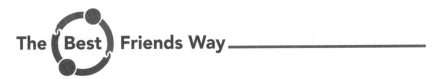

The (Best) Friends Way _____

Life Story: What type of exercise did the *person* do in the past? Has the *person* enjoyed exercising in a group environment or with others? Did anyone ever take an extended hiking trip that involved camping out?

The Arts: Take photographs along the way. Pick up pretty leaves for art projects.

Music: Sing a song as you walk.

Exercise: No matter how slow or fast the pace, this activity helps keep all individuals active.

Old Sayings: "Walk a mile in my shoes." "Slow and steady wins the race."

Old Skills: Walking is an old skill. The walking club includes other old skills, such as socializing, setting goals, planning, and organizing.

Sensory: Stop and smell the fresh flowers on your daily walk, look at birds in the trees, listen to the sounds of nature, or take a break during the walk and sit on a bench and watch the world go by.

Spirituality: Being in the sunshine not only fights depression but also puts us in touch with Mother Nature.

Early Dementia: Let *persons* use a pedometer to count their steps. They can set goals and keep track of their progress.

Late Dementia: Take the *person* who is in a wheelchair for a trip outside.

Conversation: Give a compliment while walking: "Mark, you look like you are in great shape. Have you always been athletic?" Encourage: "I know you are a bit tired, but we just have a few more minutes to go. Let's hold hands and keep moving." Sight-see: "Look at that beautiful statue in the town square. That's something to be proud of." Offer some motivation or a gentle tease: "Good morning, Teresa. Let's get moving. Your doctor wants you to walk every day to build your strength!"

An ounce of prevention . . .

Use common sense, and don't push persons beyond their capacities.

Relaxation Hour

The late afternoon can be a time when our energy lags. This activity involves simple yoga or exercise and soothing music, creating a segment of the day in the afternoon for *persons* with dementia to engage in planned relaxation.

The Basics

- A videotape about yoga or staff member who is familiar with seated yoga techniques
- A relaxing videotape/DVD or music; the violinist André Rieu's video (find on the Web) has met with great success
- Items from the activity Stop and Smell the Roses (p. 76) that evoke calm and relaxation (e.g., chamomile, lavender)

Lower the lights, if possible. For a good stretch, demonstrate sitting up straight on the edge of your chair, feet flat on the floor directly below your knees. Let your hands rest on your thighs, take a long deep breath, and exhale slowly. Inhale deeply again, reaching for the ceiling with the crown of your head, lengthening your spine. As you exhale, slide your shoulders down your back, dropping your shoulders away from your ears. After six to eight breaths, bring your arms back to your resting position and relax your back.

Next, encourage all present to engage in shoulder rolls (rolling the shoulders slowly forward and backward) and spinal rolls (bending over slowly with the face to the floor and slowly returning to a seated position). An important step is for the leader to demonstrate each move. Seeing the moves helps *persons* mimic the stretches.

Listen to violin music or other classical music after seated yoga or as a full relaxation hour. Use a diffuser to enjoy some calming scents.

Variation: Add techniques from Breathing for Health (p. 77).

Submitted by Sally Fitch, Program Manager of Events and Volunteers, Mid Coast Senior Health Center, Brunswick, ME.

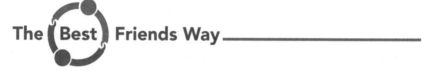

The (Best) Friends Way

Life Story: Do some gentle reminiscing during this time. Find out whether someone meditated or who in the group enjoyed relaxing/calming down. Did anyone have a particularly stressful job? How did he or she relax?

Music: Celebrate classical music during this activity.

Old Sayings: "Being mellow." "Getting off the fast track." "An apple a day keeps the doctor away." "Early to bed and early to rise makes a [man or woman] healthy, wealthy, and wise."

Sensory: The scents and aromas discussed in Stop and Smell the Roses (p. 76) go well with this activity.

Late Dementia: Hold the *person's* hand. Encourage him or her to follow the moves of the leader or just focus on the music.

Conversation: In a gentle voice: "Jasmine, how does that violin music make you feel?" Query: "Does it feel good to stretch at this time of day?" Turn a "no" into a "yes": "We've worked hard all morning, Bob. It's time for our 15-minute relaxation break!" Ask an easy question: "Cynthia, what do you do to relax when you are feeling stressed out?"

The Basics

- Handbells, four blue and four red bells per box (each plays a different note)
- Taped or live music, any type that fits the group; music with a strong beat is easier to follow (there are four CDs of specially arranged piano music by James Wagner)
- *Instructor's Booklet* and *The Bellringer's Primer* by Linda Wilson and James Wagner

[All of the above are available for purchase at www.joyandaction.com]

- Leader (staff or volunteer)

Have *persons* sit in a semicircle facing the leader. Provide a red and a blue bell for each *person*. Ask the group to follow the leader as he or she moves to the music with the bells. The moves can mimic regular chair exercises with both hands held high, hands stretched out wide, hands down by one's side, or hands down in front. You can bend over, stretch back, and turn from side to side.

No one needs a musical background to participate. Familiarity with the music and a positive, "let go" attitude is all it takes.

Training Tip: Ask staff to practice various moves for a song to present to the ringers. Instead of memorizing moves, let them flow to fit the music. This is more fun for everyone.

Submitted by Cherry Liter, ACC for Bells Exercise Workshops, Lexington, KY.

Saved by the Bell

Exercising can be more fun for all of us if it is not presented as a task to be done. *Persons* with dementia can get some great physical and mental exercise while enjoying the rhythm of bells.

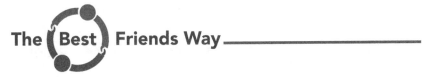

The Best Friends Way

Life Story: *Persons* usually have fond memories of music and songs. Make note of *persons'* favorite music and include a variety of music during the session. Did anyone ever ring a church bell or a dinner bell?

Exercise: Physical benefits include upper body strength, range of motion, deep breathing, and eye–hand coordination. Mental benefits include concentration, recognition of cues, and an overall sense of fun and well-being.

Humor: Laughter comes naturally listening to oom-pa-pa music, ragtime jazz on the piano, or a Broadway tune with humorous lyrics.

Sensory: Listening and moving to music, tapping toes, clapping hands, and singing wake up all of the senses.

Spirituality: This activity is great for bonding, thereby meeting a *person's* need to belong and to be valued.

Early Dementia: A *person* may like to be the leader for some music selections.

Late Dementia: Place a bell in a *person's* hand and play along with him or her.

Conversation: Share memories: "Were you ever in a band? Which instrument did you play?" Ask for a demonstration: "Sabrina, can you show us how you reach to the ceiling with both bells?" Compliment: "Ida, you are a great conductor."

A Day at the Spa

Most people enjoy being pampered and having a day of relaxation. This activity uses massage and pampering to provide lots of relaxing entertainment for the *person* with dementia.

The Basics

Set up a room as a spa. Include relaxing instrumental music, aromatherapy (see Stop and Smell the Roses, p. 76), and warm, comforting lighting. Spend the day pampering the *person* with a manicure (see Volume One, Hand Care, p. 125), a massage, a facial, and possibly a bubble bath.

Resident-to-Resident Massage
Residents are positioned in chairs or standing in a circle, allowing enough space to massage comfortably the neck, back, and arms of the *person* in front of them. Staff can participate in the circle or, depending on resident involvement, may need to demonstrate and encourage those in the circle.

Submitted by Rosemarie Harris, Director, Pinegrove of Vista Del Monte, Santa Barbara, CA.

Butter 'n Sugar Hand Treatment
- Teaspoon of butter (do not use margarine; it does not work as well)
- ½ teaspoon of sugar
- Towel
- Warm water

Place butter into the palm of the *person's* hand and sprinkle on ½ teaspoon of sugar. Work the butter and sugar throughout the hands and fingers, using a washing-type movement. Go slowly, making sure that every nook and cranny gets reached. The butter works like a great lotion to soften, and the sugar acts as an exfoliant. After a couple of minutes of massaging each other's hands, rinse in warm water and dry with a soft towel.

Submitted by Kathleen "Mimi" Taylor, Activity Director, Good Shepherd Healthcare Center, Jaffrey, NH.

Variation: Take elements of this activity for a short "spa" treatment, particularly if the *person* is having a bad day and might benefit from a positive distraction that helps him or her feel good. Small wooden rollers that make massaging someone's hands, neck, or body easier are available.

Life Story: Did the *person* enjoy spas or pampering him- or herself? Did he or she ever get massages, manicures, or pedicures or take bubble baths? Does the *person* like to be touched or prefer less physical contact?

Music: Play soft, relaxing music while giving the massage.

Exercise: Giving someone a massage exercises fine motor movements and the arms.

Old Sayings: "Rub-a-dub-dub." "Hand over hand." "Lend a hand." "Helping hand."

Old Skills: Holding and gently massaging the hands of another is a familiar old skill.

Sensory: The feel of the butter and the sugar on the hands and the pleasant smell can really invigorate the *person*!

Spirituality: The simple act of doing something for someone else can be very rewarding and provide the *person* with a sense of being needed and purposeful.

Late Dementia: A gentle massage may feel especially good to the *person* who is nonambulatory.

Conversation: Ask for an opinion: "What do you think about this wooden massager—is it better than a good old-fashioned back rub?" Reminisce: "Have you ever been to a spa and gotten a massage?" Give a choice: "Roberta, do you like this pink nail polish or this red polish?" Offer a friendly tease to encourage participation: "I know you think this is pretty silly, Mr. Thomas, but humor me; just try it for a few minutes and let me know what you think!"

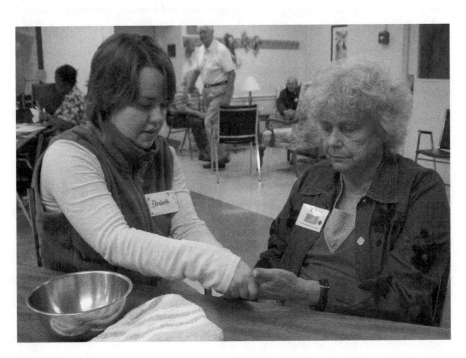

Laughter Is the Best Medicine

All human beings laugh from the beginning of life to the end of life. *Persons* with dementia can exercise this universal, physical attribute and feel better after smiling, giggling, or laughing.

The Basics

Laughter exercises are based on everyone's natural ability to laugh using three sounds and breaths. The first is "ho" from center (stomach), then "ha" from the chest (heart), and "hee" from the smile (neck and face). Before leading the activity, become familiar with some examples of ways to get the group laughing, such as laughing as you say the vowels, laughing a tune instead of singing the words, or mimicking a penguin walking. For a list of ideas, refer to the Web site listed below.

Gather the group into a circle. Discuss some of the things that make people laugh, the benefits of laughter, and laughing just for fun. For the laughter exercises, *persons* can be seated or standing in a circle.

Begin this laughing exercise activity with a greeting, such as "Aloha," and a laugh, "Ha, ha, ha!" Introduce various examples of laughter exercises (noted above), then add new ones as the laughter exercises continue. At the end of each exercise, clap hands and laugh, "Ho, ho, ha, ha, ha." Repeat three times. Conclude the activity by discussing positive aspects of laughter.

Submitted by Cherry Liter, Certified Laughter Leader (CLL), Lexington, KY. For information on Laughter Club workshops, go to www.worldlaughtertour.com.

The 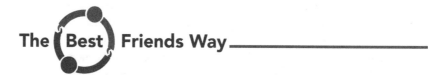 Friends Way

Life Story: Use examples from *persons'* life stories for ideas for laughter, such as funny stories about children or pets, old jokes, and old fashion "disasters," such as bell-bottom pants or prom dresses. Does anyone have a funny story to share?

Exercise: Laughing is a full-body exercise: Internal organs jog, the heart pumps fresh oxygen, brain chemistry changes, and stress is relieved naturally.

Old Skills: Feel the laughter while giving a friend a shoulder rub.

Sensory: Joy comes when *persons* hear the laughter and see the funny poses of others.

Early Dementia: Ask *persons* to lead certain exercises.

Late Dementia: Laughing to the lyrics of songs instead of singing the words may be funny to *persons*. Some *persons* may laugh simply because laughter is contagious.

Conversation: Share memories: "Darrell, did you ever laugh until you cried?" Ask for help: "Virginia, how might a lion roar?" Compliment: "Joe, your laugh is contagious." Ask for opinions: "Do you like hearty laughs or softer laughs?" or "Do you feel better after laughing?"

The Basics

Choose music with a good rhythm or beat that is easy to follow. Begin with inviting one or two *persons* to stand and join hands with you, and encourage others to sway and move to the music. *Persons* who are nonambulatory enjoy movement while still seated. Gently encourage everyone to "give it a try." Sometimes those you least expect to participate have the most fun.

Variations: To celebrate springtime or May Day, dance a modified Maypole Dance, inside or outdoors. The maypole is a pole that is decorated with streamers that those who are celebrating hold while dancing. In addition to the English Maypole tradition, Maypoles are enduring spring traditions in the Czech Republic, Slovakia, Finland, Sweden, Germany, Austria, and India. Invite *persons* to form a circle around the Maypole and pick up one of the colorful streamers. As the music is played, have everyone move in a rhythmic way to the right or the left holding onto a streamer. This movement to the music will eventually combine the streamers into a multicolored braid.

Another variation is to watch one of the new celebrity "dance competition" shows on television. Many will enjoy the humor and positive energy of the show.

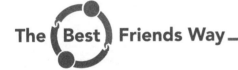 The (Best) Friends Way

Life Story: Has anyone danced the polka, a square dance, or a line dance? Maybe someone has participated in dance inspired from other countries, such as dancing the Irish jig. Does anyone know how to fiddle?

Music: Vary the music to have different tempos depending on the group. *Persons* who choose not to dance may simply enjoy the music.

Exercise: Dancing, whether it is fast or slow, provides excellent exercise.

Humor: Part of the fun of movement to music is the socialization experience. Comments should be designed to bring joy and laughter, such as "We should take this show on the road" or "If we were any better, we would have to charge admission."

Old Sayings: "I could have danced all night." "Got on my dancing shoes."

Sensory: The beat of the music and the touch of another's hand stir the senses.

Conversation: Encourage: "Jake, we have a spot right here for you." Tease: "Sabrina, I'll bet you were the best dancer in Charlestown when you were in college there." Reminisce: "Jake, did you have school dances when you were in high school in Kansas City?" Ask for help: "Robert, would you show me that step one more time?"

Group Dancing

Dancing is an old skill that many find pleasurable and nostalgic. *Persons* with dementia may be more motivated to join in when they see others having a good time at this dance group.

An ounce of prevention . . .

Some persons are excellent dancers and are too active for some partners. Group dancing tends to solve this concern. Watch for instability of all persons, and space staff strategically. Be sensitive to those who have a tradition of not dancing because of religious beliefs.

Stop and Smell the Roses

We've all enjoyed aromas and perfume, including the smell of freshly baked bread, the scent of clean linen, and the fragrance of a bouquet of roses. Many programs have their own versions of aromatherapy and are discovering the benefits of using scents for therapeutic effect for *persons* with dementia.

The Basics

Choose a specific scent for the session. There are dozens, if not hundreds, of potential scents, but to start, focus on more common scents: lavender, mint, eucalyptus, vanilla, orange, lemon, or anise (like licorice). Look for inexpensive hand lotions or candles with these scents, or go to a specialty store that has essential oils. Other items with nice scents include soaps, bath salts, various herbal teas, flowers, and herbs (e.g., rosemary, mint leaves, lavender).

Choose a comfortable environment, with lights dim and soft music playing. Candles of the same fragrance, bath salts, and lotions are used for each session to help the *person* identify the aroma. Some *persons* may enjoy a foot bath using the bath salts, whereas others enjoy having lotions applied to their legs and arms.

Use the scents in a relaxing way while discussing their properties. Some common beliefs are that lavender is for relaxation, chamomile for calm, rosemary for memory, eucalyptus for energy, and so forth.

Submitted by Rosemarie Harris, Director, Pinegrove of Vista Del Monte, Santa Barbara, CA.

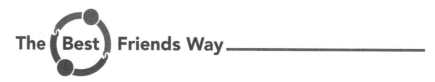

The Best Friends Way

Life Story: Does anyone recall having an herb garden? Did anyone in the group make sachets or grow flowers in his or her garden? Who likes perfume or cologne? Did anyone practice herbal medicine?

The Arts: After enjoying a bouquet, press and dry flowers and herbs for a variety of art projects. Make clove oranges (see Volume One, Oranges with Cloves, p. 91).

Exercise: Walk outside to experience natural scents and smells in a spring garden.

Sensory: The sense of smell is one that triggers memory for a long period of time. Buy a bread machine and use it daily.

Spirituality: In some faiths, aroma plays a part in religious services (e.g., incense).

Early Dementia: Engage *persons* in a discussion about the value of aromatherapy, and invite them to pick a scent to smell.

Late Dementia: Encourage the *person* to crush a lavender or rosemary plant in his or her fingers and smell it (or do it in your own fingers and let him or her smell the lovely aroma).

Conversation: Brainstorm: "What does this vanilla scent remind you of?" Reminisce: "Have you ever smelled eucalyptus trees?" Vote: "Which of these scents do you like best?" Make a connection: "Raymond, I love my trips to Florida. Were you ever there when the orange trees were blooming?"

The Basics

Breath-Counting Exercise: Encourage each *person* in the group to find a comfortable position for sitting upright, with arms and legs uncrossed and, if possible, feet flat on the floor. Make sure that everyone is as comfortable as possible. Exhale completely through the mouth, making a "whoosh" sound. Then close your mouth and inhale slowly through your nose to a count of four. Pause for a moment, as if holding your breath, for a count of one. Then exhale completely through your mouth, making a "whoosh" sound to a count of six. This is one breath. Repeat the cycle for a total of five breaths. To end this session, take a deep breath and stretch your arms and legs as if waking from a short nap. This exercise gains in power with repetition and practice.

Energizing Breathing Exercise: Encourage everyone present to sit in a comfortable, upright position with his or her spine straight. With your mouth gently closed, breathe in and out of your nose in a short but quick manner. Feel the breath reach the belly and then into the chest. To give an idea of how this is done, think of someone using a bellows or bicycle pump. The up stroke is inhalation, the down stroke is exhalation. Both are equal in length.

The rate of breathing should be consistent but a bit more rapid than usual. Repeat the breath four to five times, and then breathe normally again. This exercise, also called the stimulating breath, can be used during times of fatigue to awaken from feelings of tiredness. It uses short, fast, rhythmic breaths to increase energy.

Submitted by Jim Concotelli, PhD, Vice-President of Resident Programs, Horizon Bay Senior Communities, Tampa, FL.

Breathing for Health

We all breathe to maintain life, yet many spiritual healers believe that conscious breathing can contribute to good health. *Persons* with dementia may enjoy and benefit from this breathing exercise.

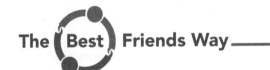 The **Best** Friends Way

Life Story: Who has liked to relax, and who stays busy all the time? Did anyone in the group ever practice meditation?

Music: Music can accompany this activity if it is soft and without lyrics.

Exercise: The lungs get a good workout, and this activity supports good posture.

Old Sayings: "Don't waste your breath!" "Don't hold your breath." "Breath of life." "Out of breath."

Sensory: Feel your breath as it enters and leaves your body.

Late Dementia: This is an exercise that many persons can accomplish with a bit of modeling and conversation.

Conversation: Don't converse much during the actual exercise, but beforehand say, "Michelle, Eric, and Ted, please join us for an exercise class. This one is easy because we all take good breaths of air each minute!" Educate: "Many spiritual leaders say that breath exercises help us stay healthy. I feel better already."

Celebration of Life

This activity involves a musical party with lots of sound, rhythm, and props for play. It creates excitement, validation, and positive emotions that last throughout the day for *persons* with dementia. It was created to empower residents not just to be entertained, but also to be entertainers themselves.

The Basics

Put an hour aside for a group musical celebration. Go to a party store to buy props, including silly plastic party hats of all shapes and colors, feather boas, plastic jewelry, and so forth. Buy some plastic shakers, maracas, or other handheld percussion instruments, such as tambourines. The facilitator should purchase a small djembe—an African-style drum (Remo Drum Company makes an affordable version that can be purchased at your local music store or on the Internet). Inflatable guitars produce smiles and are great props.

You will need a portable boom box to play the music. Compile a song list that will excite and touch the residents' hearts. Good songs include

"Amore" by Dean Martin (celebrates Italian heritage)

"Rock Around the Clock" by Bill Haley & The Comets

"Blue Suede Shoes" by Elvis Presley

"She Loves You" by The Beatles

"These Boots Are Made for Walking" by Nancy Sinatra

"Danny Boy" (any version; celebrates Irish heritage)

"All Shook Up" by Elvis Presley

"Happy Trails" by Roy Rogers

"Roll Out the Barrel" (any version; celebrates Polish heritage)

"Working in a Coal Mine"

"Hot Hot Hot" (any version; celebrates Latin heritage)

Enlist staff to volunteer in the celebration. Seat the participants in a large circle, approximately an arm's length apart, with plenty of room in the middle for performing, dancing, and singing. Have the facilitator introduce each song, tie it to life stories when appropriate, and beat the drum with a steady beat to keep the group momentum going.

Create a 1-hour program of music with celebration, including raising the American flag during patriotic songs, giving residents an inflatable guitar to play, having dancing puppets, and encouraging group participation with the maracas or other hand rhythm instruments. Start with some slower songs and build momentum with faster music.

Encourage dancing among the residents and staff. At some point, try singing along to "Danny Boy;" it often brings some tears, but it is okay for residents to cry from happy memories. Make a patriotic song a high-light of the event with American flags. Wind down with a quieter song, such as "Happy Trails." Take time when appropriate to reminisce about the topic (e.g., baseball games with "Take Me Out to the Ball Game").

Very Important: Don't be afraid to be rambunctious and loud and have some fun. This is a party! Serve refreshments after the program, not during.

Submitted by David Currier, Alzheimer's Program Director, Winship Green Nursing and Rehabilitation Center, Bath, ME.

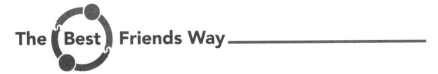

The (Best) Friends Way

Life Story: Who always enjoyed a fun party? Has anyone ever been in a band or marched in a parade? Who enjoys listening to band music with lots of drumming? Who thinks that they do not have any rhythm? Has someone always wanted to be a drummer? Who liked celebrations?

The Arts: Collect as many different types of drums or ways of drumming as pos-sible for discussion. Study the intricate designs on some drums.

Music: This activity is all about making music and is for everyone—the musical and the nonmusical *person* alike.

Exercise: This activity encourages upper body movement and dance.

Old Sayings: "Marching to the beat of a different drummer." "Party animal." "The Life of the party."

Sensory: The program serves as a vehicle to laugh, reminisce, celebrate fond memories, and connect with neighbors as well as providing tactile/sensory stimulation.

Late Dementia: Most *persons* like to keep time to the beat of a drum.

Conversation: Make a connection: "Juanita, you are from Mexico. This next song is from Mexico, too, and I'm playing it in your honor." Share something in common: "Dr. Zechman, I have just learned that you were in a drum and bugle corps while in the army, and so was I." Encourage conversation: "Did any of you watch Ed Sullivan and see The Beatles perform on his show?"

Guided Relaxation

Many individuals have found that a guided relaxation exercise, with descriptive and soothing words and images, has the power to transform our day. *Persons* with dementia also benefit from this soothing activity.

The Basics

In this script (see facing page), which lasts a recommended 15 to 20 minutes, participants take an imaginary journey along a beach, listening to the birds and waves, and watching a brilliant sunset. Play soft instrumental music, nature sounds, or classical music in the background. Read the script slowly, pause after each sentence, and use a soft and soothing voice. Use the script as an inspiration and model to write your own relaxation exercises.

Submitted by Jim Concotelli, PhD, Vice-President of Resident Programs, Horizon Bay Senior Communities, Tampa, FL.

The 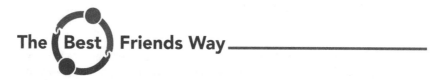 Best Friends Way

Life Story: Younger *persons* may be somewhat familiar with this newer method of relaxation, but for others it will be a totally new experience. What do *persons* do for relaxation? Did anyone have a personal trainer or belong to a health club?

The Arts: A famous painting could be the focal point of the guided meditation.

Music: Play soft classical music in the background or music selections that involve natural sounds.

Exercise: Although a small part of this activity, there is stretching and deep breathing, both of which are physically rewarding.

Sensory: *Persons* take an imaginary trip along the beach and relive the sights and sounds. They listen to a soft and soothing voice as the script unfolds.

Spirituality: Even though this activity involves an imaginary ocean scene, it can evoke the feeling of the spiritual in the *person's* created world.

Early Dementia: *Persons* with early dementia, especially *persons* who are younger in age, will be very much in tune with this activity.

Conversation: Laugh together: "Selma, I almost went to sleep during that quiet time, and I looked at you and you were all but snoring yourself. That relaxation really worked for us." Reminisce: "Elaine, did you ever count sheep when you were trying to go to sleep?" Have a thoughtful reflection: "Isn't it good that we have interesting ways now to help us relax? We live in such a busy world." Encourage conversation: "Bill, did you and your family spend much time on the beach when you lived in Seattle?"

A Walk on the Beach at Sunset (Guided Relaxation Script)

Allow yourself to be as comfortable as possible. Close your eyes and become aware of which parts of your body are feeling tense and which parts are relaxed.

Take a few slow, deep breaths, taking the air in through your nose, holding it momentarily, and then slowly exhaling through your nose. With each exhale, allow yourself to calm. Each time you exhale, say "relax."

Take the air in and let the air out, allowing yourself to relax . . . relax . . . relax. Inhale . . . calm. Exhale . . . relax. (Pause for 2 to 3 minutes; allow the group to deepen their relaxation.)

In a few moments, I am going to describe a very vivid scene in which you will picture yourself walking along a beach. I want you to imagine this scene as though you were there experiencing not only the sights but also the sounds, smells, tastes, and touches.

Imagine that it is a bright summer day. You decide to go for a walk along the beach. The sun is radiating warmth and comfort as it shines boldly. The sky is crystal clear without a cloud in sight. The grains of sand beneath your feet shine from the sunlight and warm the soles of your feet. The sound of the waves beating against the shore echoes in the air. You feel the warm, light breeze brush up against your face as you walk slowly along the beach.

Far off in the distance, you hear the cries of sea gulls. You watch them glide through the sky, swoop down into the sea, and then fly off again.

The waves are gliding in . . . and the waves are gliding out. You feel more and more calm. Continue to watch the waves glide in . . . and out.

As you walk farther along the shore, you decide to rest. As you sit down, you feel the pure white sand and gaze out to the sea, staring intently at the rhythmic, methodical motion of the waves rolling into shore.

Each wave breaks against the coast and rises slowly upward along the beach, leaving a fan of white foam. It retreats back out to sea, only to be replaced by another wave that crashes against the shore . . . works its way up the beach . . . then slowly retreats out to sea.

With each motion of the wave as it glides in and out, you find yourself feeling more and more relaxed, more and more calm . . . more and more serene.

Now as you stare off into the distance, you see that the sun is beginning to sink into the horizon. The sun is sinking down, and you feel more and more relaxed as you see its movement going down . . . down . . . down.

The sky is turning brilliant colors of red . . . orange . . . yellow . . . green . . . blue . . . and purple. As the sun sets, sinking down . . . down . . . down . . . into the horizon, you feel very relaxed and soothed. You watch the sun as it sinks down . . . down . . . down.

The beating of the waves, the smell and the taste of the sea, the salt, the cries of the gulls, the warmth against your body—all of these sights, sounds, and smells leave you feeling soothed, very calm, very serene.

And you relax . . . relax . . . relax.

For the next 5 to 10 minutes, allow yourself to enjoy this state of deep relaxation. When you notice your mind drifting to thoughts of everyday life, recall the sounds of the waves rolling in and out and enjoy the sights and sounds of the beach.

(Pause and allow the group 5 to 10 minutes for silent relaxation.)

In a few moments, I will count to help you awaken from your deep relaxation. When I reach the count of 5, your eyes will open and you will feel completely refreshed and totally relaxed. Begin by taking a few deep breaths to awaken yourself.

1 . . . 2 . . . 3 . . . 4 . . . 5. Now take one last deep breath and, as you inhale, stretch your arms out as you would after a short nap. Feel yourself awakening, refreshed, relaxed, and ready for the rest of your day. (Repeat these last instructions until everyone is alert.)

Tai Chi

Tai Chi Chuan, commonly called Tai Chi, is a Chinese martial art that is associated with good health and longevity. It emphasizes the use of the mind to coordinate the relaxed body, as opposed to the use of brute strength. This activity has become popular in many long-term care programs for *persons* with dementia, who relate to its simple movement and peacefulness.

The Basics

Tai Chi emphasizes breathing and movement that are both flowing and graceful. Following is a sample Tai Chi exercise called Moving the Chi Ball:

> From a standing position, lift your hands and arms in front of your belly area as if holding a small beach ball. Shift your hands and arms to the right as you shift your weight to the right. Lift your hands and arms up to chest height as you circle them in front of your body and to the left side. Shift your weight to the left as well. Continue to circle your arms and shift your weight from side to side. The breath matches the movement: Inhale on the upward movement of the hands and arms to the right, and exhale on the movement to the left and downward. After 8 to 10 movements, reverse the direction of the circle.

Tip: The activity is easily modified for *persons* who cannot stand.

Submitted by Jim Concotelli, PhD, Vice-President of Resident Programs, Horizon Bay Senior Communities, Tampa, FL.

The 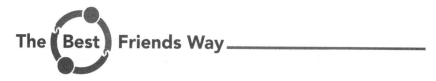 Best Friends Way

Life Story: Did any *persons* grow up exercising using the Tai Chi method? Are any *persons* from countries such as China and Japan, where this art is practiced widely? Who is eager to try new things? Did anyone make exercise a daily ritual?

Music: Exercise to some slow, soft music.

Exercise: Tai Chi is low impact and therefore safe for most *persons*. It promotes valuable stretching.

Sensory: Feel the stretching and listen to the groans as the muscles resist being challenged. Enjoy watching the group learn a new form of exercise.

Spirituality: Tai Chi has often been referred to as "meditation in motion."

Early Dementia: Some *persons* may be very familiar with Tai Chi and be able to lead the group in the moves, or they may enjoy reading a statement about the meaning of the words *Tai Chi*. They may also be interested in beginning or continuing a class in Tai Chi in the community.

Conversation: Encourage interaction: "Judy, when you were in Tokyo, did you see people in the parks early in the morning doing Tai Chi?" Laugh together: "Mr. Roberson, did you ever think that you would work this hard and actually have fun?" Ponder: "I wonder why it took so long for exercises like this one to catch on in the United States."

The Basics _____

There are many varieties of exercise bands (large rubber bands or straps). From the Web or from any sports store (Internet search words: resistance bands) purchase a band for each person who will be participating. See also a good discussion on how to buy bands at exercise.about.com/cs/exerciseworkouts/a/resistance_2.htm.

    The following are a few of the basic moves that can be done using the stretch bands. These exercises can be done sitting or standing.

1. Grasp both ends of the band so that the length of the band is shoulder-width apart. Raise the band over the head. First, slowly stretch your right arm to the side about 6 to 12 inches (above shoulder level) and repeat the stretch with the left arm. Repeat 10 times on each side.

2. Place the band on your back, with the ends under the arms. Grip the band ends with each hand in front of the underarms. Press the arms forward. Pause and slowly return to the starting position. Repeat 10 times.

3. Step on the band with the right foot, curl the end of the band around the right hand, and slowly curl the wrist upward toward your body; repeat on the left side. Repeat 10 times on each side.

    There are many variations of the above. Have the group create its own exercise program.

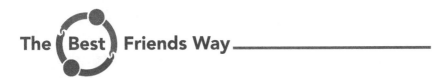

The (Best) Friends Way _____

Life Story: Has anyone lifted weights? Did he or she do calisthenics in the army? Is anyone an "exercise buff?" Has anyone worked in jobs where a lot of muscle was required to do heavy lifting?

Humor: Laugh about how funny it would be to see a cat stretching with one of the bands.

Old Skills: Many *persons* have been in jobs demanding heavy lifting.

Old Sayings: "Pulling your own weight." "Use it or lose it."

Spirituality: The body is spoken of as the temple of the spirit in the writings of the Christian faith.

Early Dementia: Encourage membership in an exercise class.

Conversation: Reminisce: "Otto, I'll bet your strength came in handy when you were a policeman in New York." Encourage: "Julie, did you use this kind of exercise when you were the athletic director at West Side Elementary School?" Recall a famous figure: "Darnell, did you ever watch Jack LaLanne do exercises on television or see his ads selling juicers?"

Strength Training

The "baby boomers" have made physical fitness a priority, spending time at the gym and lifting weights. Many *persons* with dementia, especially those who are younger, will enjoy this strength training exercise using inexpensive elastic bands.

An ounce of prevention . . .

Start slowly for persons who have never used bands for stretching, and gradually add more exercises. Check to determine if the exercise is not appropriate for some persons.

Adult Education

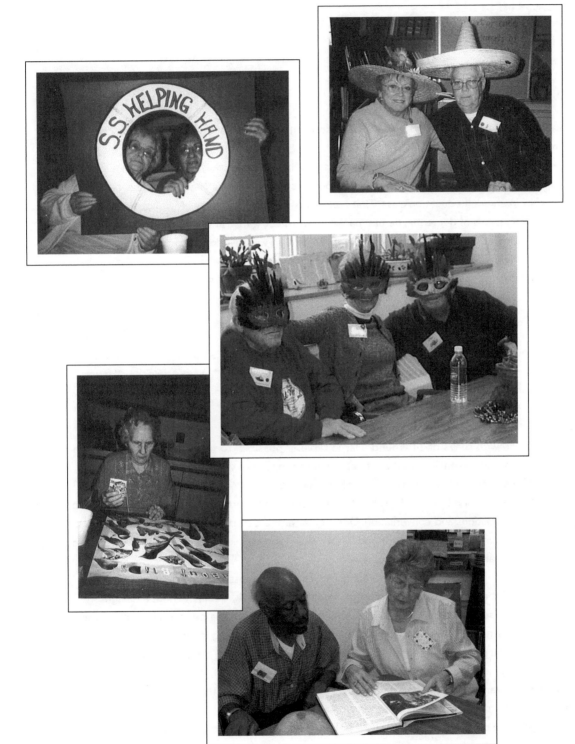

Adult Education

Re-creating the classroom experience can be fascinating and rewarding in a dementia care environment. Learning is a long-held skill; almost everyone has had some experience with the classroom during his or her life. At first, the reader may think that this does not make much sense in a dementia care environment; conventional wisdom is that *persons* with dementia cannot learn new material such as that taught in an adult education class. That concept is changing, as James McKillop noted in Chapter 1; despite his diagnosis of dementia, he has learned how to use e-mail and new digital cameras. We have found that offering a short class or discussion on an interesting topic works well. It seems that *persons* still enjoy the *experience* of learning, even if they may not be able to retain all of the material discussed.

An added benefit of the activities in this chapter is that staff and *persons* can learn together. In addition, younger staff members benefit from the wisdom of their elders; many *persons* with dementia still recall interesting or historic events through which they have lived.

When you teach the class, begin with some information about the topic or use trivia (fun, short facts) that can be revealed or formed into questions. For example, if you were doing trivia about musical legends, then you could talk about some of Elvis Presley's No. 1 hits (e.g., "Jailhouse Rock," "Hound Dog") or recall his middle name (Aaron). You can ask what Frank Sinatra's nickname was (Ol' Blue Eyes) or where he was born (Hoboken, NJ).

To promote successful group or classroom activities:

- Create a circle with chairs or sit around a large table, if possible, to foster closeness and re-create a classroom experience. Small groups are best, but larger ones can work.
- Use one of the topics in this chapter, or develop your own!
- Have the group leader introduce the subject, pass around any appropriate objects, and lead the group in some trivia questions and conversation. Don't be afraid to be provocative; a question such as, "Is it a good idea to lend money to close friends?" or "How long should you know each other before getting married?" can evoke a good discussion.
- Incorporate each *person's* life story into the topics as much as possible.
- Stimulate all of the senses: Bring in items that involve taste, touch, smell, hearing, and sight.
- Don't make the session too lengthy—approximately 30 to 45 minutes per class or topic. Even if you find lots of information or items to share, you need not use everything in one session.
- Be flexible. If you plan a topic and the group goes in another direction, then just go with them! You can always do the planned topic at another time.
- Be prepared. Even a short amount of time spent researching topics in the library, at a bookstore, or on the Internet will make everything go better.
- Encourage some participants to read aloud or help plan or implement the group activity.

- Have at least two staff members present. If someone wants to leave, then do your best to encourage him or her to participate, but it is okay if the *person* wants to watch from the sidelines!
- Consider creating a class topic committee to plan group activities and research and write future topics (see Chapter 9, Planning Group, p. 163).

We draw your attention to a few specific activities in this chapter:

Lunar New Year (p. 89), Hanukkah (p. 108), Maple Harvest (p. 109), and Oktoberfest (p. 97) all are examples of activities that celebrate a particular region or heritage. Use these as models for a relevant classroom topic for your group.

Touring Mexico (p. 101) may help a *person* who misses travel. He or she may no longer be able to take an actual cruise or get on an 8-hour flight, but an activity such as this encourages flights of imagination.

Give Me Five! (p. 107) is a clever activity that uses the number 5 and is an example of an activity that may not need much research ahead of time.

Note: Most of these activities can be adapted for one-to-one times.

Tips for Staff Training: Model these classroom activities ahead of time for staff. It will be fun, staff will learn more about one another, and it will encourage everyone to think about the importance of lifelong learning.

CHAPTER SIX ACTIVITIES

The Basics

Before Class: Research the Lunar New Year Celebration. The date varies by year but most of the time falls around the end of January into mid-February. Check a calendar for the exact dates each year. The celebration lasts for 7 days, with the first day being of the utmost importance for the kick-off celebration. Gather items from local ethnic stores celebrating the New Year, purchase or prepare Asian food, get Asian-themed music CDs, consider renting a movie or documentary featuring the holiday, and develop art projects related to the theme, such as a papier mâché dragon.

Also, note the animal that symbolizes the year by incorporating it into crafts and décor. Is it the year of the rooster, rat, or tiger?

At Class Time: Introduce the topic with some music, share trivia, do an art project, offer a New Year's toast, and wind down with an Asian-themed dessert and herbal tea. If your program is in a city with a large Asian population, take an appropriate group to a parade or invite a youth group in to perform traditional dances.

Submitted by Tammie Nguyen, Program Director, Catholic Charities, San Jose, CA.

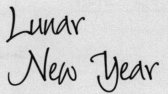

Lunar New Year

The Lunar New Year is celebrated on the first day of the lunar calendar by most Asian communities (colloquially called the "Chinese New Year"). It marks a new "beginning," and is celebrated with new clothing and an eclectic array of food offered by families and friends. It is one of the most important days in Asian communities and will arouse memories of the sights, sounds, aromas, and high-spirited feeling of this special time for *persons* with dementia.

The 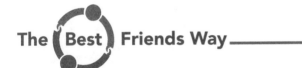 Best Friends Way

Life Story: Has the *person* celebrated the Lunar New Year throughout his or her life? Has the *person* traveled to Vietnam or China? What are the *person's* childhood memories of the Lunar New Year celebration? Has anyone lived in a city with a large Asian population (e.g., Seattle, Vancouver, San Francisco) and thus is familiar with the New Year's parade or celebration?

The Arts: Create a papier mâché animal head for the parade. Create a "firecracker" decoration by covering an empty toilet paper roll with strips of red construction paper. String the firecrackers together using yarn, and hang it in the doorway.

Music: Bring in sounds of cultural music to celebrate the new year, and keep time to the music.

Exercise: Enjoy a parade using the papier mâché animal head made by the group.

Old Skills: Preparing food and decorations for the celebration may draw on old skills.

Continued on next page

Continued from previous page

Sensory: Red is the color of choice to symbolize the good fortune for the new year. Another way to provide décor is to have cherry blossom flowers in a large vase because this is the flower of the new year. Serve food that is associated with the Lunar New Year, such as sticky rice cakes or trays of various sweet fruit treats.

Spirituality: Good fortune, prosperity, and health are basic greetings to one another at the start of the new year. These are symbolized by offerings of food, gifts of money (called *li xi* in red envelopes), and visitation to temples.

Early Dementia: Invite the *person* to help research information on the Lunar New Year and present it to the group. Go out for Chinese, Vietnamese, or Thai food!

Late Dementia: The sights and sounds are stimulating.

Conversation: Ask with humor: "Did you get rich from your red envelope?" Reminisce: "Did you shoot off firecrackers to celebrate the new year?" Dream a bit: "I'd love to visit the Great Wall of China. Have you ever been to the Great Wall of China?"

The Basics ─────────────────

Before Class: Collect information and trivia about the 1950s, including fashion trends, major news events, music, and lifestyles. Visit a vintage clothing store and borrow some clothes from the 1950s. Research the 1950s on the Internet using keywords: 1950s, poodle skirts, saddle oxfords, and "sock hops." Also, gather items from the 1950s: old appliances, recordings of old radio or television shows (e.g., "American Bandstand" with Dick Clark), a poodle skirt, pictures of 1950s life, and a newspaper.

At Class Time: Pass around the items and talk about life in the 1950s. How is life different today from then? Play "Name that Tune" with music from the 1950s. Compilation CDs of early Motown recording stars are available, and satellite radio stations have channels that are dedicated to the 1950s. Once the class has guessed the tune, you might just have a spontaneous sing-along! Have a style show with the fashions from the 1950s. Talk about all of the different hairstyles: flat top, beehive, and pony tails. Discuss television shows from the era, such as *Leave It to Beaver*, *I Love Lucy*, and *The Tonight Show* with Jack Paar.

1950s

The decade of the 1950s was rich with great music, new-found freedoms, fashion, and news. *Persons* with dementia may enjoy reminiscing about life in the 1950s.

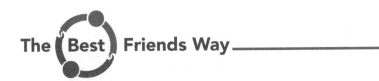

The (Best) Friends Way ─────────────────

Life Story: Who grew up in the 1950s? Where did people grow up? How was life different in the 1950s? What were the values of that time, and how have they affected the *person*? Did the *person* buy an Edsel automobile from that era or throw Frisbees, first invented in 1957?

The Arts: Make up a Burma Shave slogan.

Music: Name any popular singers from this decade and their songs ("That'll Be the Day," by The Crickets; "Jailhouse Rock," by Elvis Presley; "Lucille," by Little Richard; and "Wake Up Little Susie," by The Everly Brothers). Check the Internet for the top 10 lists of songs for each year; see how many *persons* remember the songs.

Exercise: Encourage the dancers in your group to give everyone lessons on the "Jitter Bug." Do group exercises to the music of the decade.

Humor: Sing Little Richard's "Tutti Fruitti" and laugh about the funny lyrics.

Old Sayings: "See the USA in a Chevrolet."

Early Dementia: Have a *person* model a poodle skirt or letterman's jacket.

Conversation: Reminisce: "Brad, did you like to roller skate?" Debate: "Do you think life was easier now or then?" Take a poll: "What kind of car did you drive in the 1950s?" Discuss the presidents of this era (see Hail to the Chief, p. 98). Celebrate the life story: "Jean, did you have a pair of saddle oxfords [shoes] when you were a teenager?"

Timepieces

Clocks and timepieces date back to ancient times and are a fascinating topic for many individuals. *Persons* with dementia may enjoy exploring different timepieces, from a fine watch to a German cuckoo clock.

The Basics —————————————————

Before Class: Gather a variety of timepieces (try to find as many unique and interesting pieces as possible). Research clock making and history regarding time (standard time, daylight savings time). Research clocks on the Internet using keywords: clocks, clock making, and daylight savings time.

At Class Time: Share information regarding clock making and history regarding time to spark discussion. Discuss how people told time before the invention of clocks. Discuss unusual clocks, such as sundials, Stonehenge, Big Ben, and other timepieces (e.g., church bells, factory whistle, rooster crowing), as well as clock making. Share memories of counting down time for New Year's Eve.

Show the various timepieces to the group and discuss each one. Set a cuckoo clock to go off for everyone to enjoy.

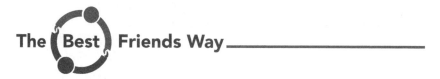

The (Best) Friends Way —————————————

Life Story: Was the *person* a collector of clocks? Find clocks that tap into the life story, such as a clock for golfers or teachers. Did anyone have a pocket watch? Did anyone buy a grandmother or grandfather clock in Germany during their military service? Did anyone ever see the outdoor flower clock in Holland, Michigan?

The Arts: Some clocks can be used as art pieces. Collect unique artistic styles of clocks.

Music: Some clocks play music. Sing "My Grandfather's Clock."

Humor: Make a joke: "That cuckoo clock is making me cuckoo!"

Old Sayings: "Time flies when you're having fun." "Spring forward, fall back." "Father Time." "Clock-in." "Time on your hands."

Old Skills: Check the time of day with the group to see if everyone's watches are running slow or fast or just right!

Sensory: Listening to the tick-tock of the timepieces can be soothing.

Spirituality: Read Ecclesiastes 3:1 from the Bible: "For everything there is a season, and a time for every purpose under heaven. . . ." Discuss the meaning of these words.

Early Dementia: Ask the *person* to read some facts from the research on clocks.

Conversation: Speculate: "Margo, why do you think we have daylight savings time?" Explore history: "Who invented cuckoo clocks? Why do you think they chose to make a clock that cuckoos?" Celebrate the life story: "Bill, you have a large collection of clocks. Tell me about them." Ask for advice: "Do you think the Swiss make the best watches?"

The Basics ────────────

Before Class: Bring in items that were created through needlework: a hand-knit sweater, an afghan, a crocheted placemat or handkerchief with a crocheted border, a needlepoint picture, or belt. Collect items used for needlework to show, such as knitting needles, embroidery hooks, balls of yarn, and embroidery hoops.

At Class Time: Many *persons* may still be able to knit and do basic sewing or needlework. They can work on their own, teach others, or demonstrate their skill to the group.

Enjoy looking together at how each item was made. Invite someone to demonstrate to the group how to knit.

Variation: Form a sewing group. Complete a project for charity, such as baby blankets for a shelter or scarves for the homeless.

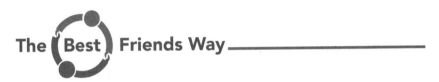

The (Best) Friends Way ────────────

Life Story: Has the *person* enjoyed doing needlework? Bring in pieces that the *person* has completed to look at and enjoy. Did he or she sew? Did anyone have a favorite hand-knitted blanket as a child? Who has a memory of a mother who was always making something?

The Arts: Create a wall hanging from fabric remnants that can be sewn together to decorate the *person's* room or the gathering room.

Exercise: Needlework is great exercise for fine motor skills.

Old Sayings: "Knit and pearl." "Tied up in a knot." "A stitch in time saves nine."

Old Skills: Quilting, crocheting, knitting, embroidery, and tatting are old skills for many *persons.*

Sensory: Running one's fingers across a needlepoint picture can provide a sensory experience.

Spirituality: Many faith communities have beautiful handmade vestments, needlepoint kneeling benches, and wall hangings. Some *persons* may enjoy looking at pictures and discussing their particular memories.

Early Dementia: Encourage the *person* to continue his or her craft by beginning a needlework project; provide assistance if needed.

Late Dementia: Place a soft, warm afghan on the *person's* lap to enjoy feeling it, and talk about the colors. Ask a *person* to rewind a ball of yarn.

Needlework

Many people have enjoyed the craft of needlework. *Persons* with dementia will enjoy looking at finished pieces and reminiscing about their craft.

Continued on next page

Continued from previous page

Conversation: Reminisce: "Loretta, how did you learn to needlepoint?" Ask for information: "Gladys, what is the difference between knitting and crocheting?" Ponder together: "Ronald, look at this monogram. I wonder what the initials BTC stand for." Reminisce: "Have you ever been to a castle where they have tapestries on the wall?"

My scissors snip and slash and slip
The needle in and out and up and down
Colors mix and stir and ramble
Patterns weave and merge and shock
The fabrics feel so soft and smooth
They smell of sizing, soap or clean
The gentle purr of my old machine
The swish and tug as my fingers pull and push and turn and twist
Every aspect of my quilting
Gives me joy to see, hear, smell, and feel
My stack of fabric neatly folded beckons me
No housework today!

Marilyn Truscott, a person with early dementia featured in the Introduction, shares a poem with us about her love of quilting, May 2003.

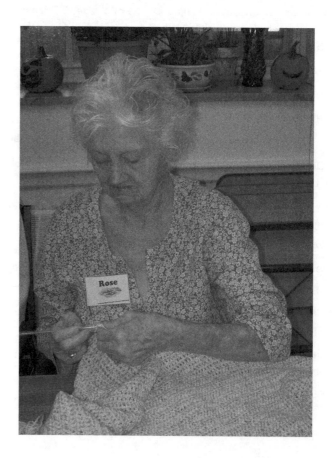

The Basics _____

Before Class: Gather pictures depicting horses and horse racing. Bring in items related to horse racing: a saddle, jockey silks, derby hat, and a mint julep cup. Research information on the history of horse racing, such as famous horses, jockeys, horse breeds, and famous horse races.

At Class Time: While looking at the items, discuss horse racing history and current events. Talk about the fashions of horse racing events. Enjoy a drink with a sprig of mint to toast the winning horse.

Variation: Develop your own horse race game. Make a track on poster board, marked off in segments. Use paper cut out horses to move along the track. Ask trivia questions or roll the dice to move forward on the track.

A Day at the Races

Horse races can be a fun and exciting activity. There is often something for everyone: the fashions, the horses, the food, or the competition! This activity brings the excitement and atmosphere of the races to *persons* with dementia.

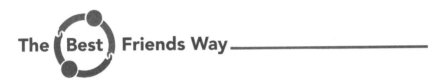

The (Best) Friends Way _____

Life Story: Has the *person* owned or ridden horses? Did the *person* enjoy attending horse races? Did the *person* grow up in "horse country"? Does he or she recall watching the Kentucky Derby on television? Did anyone bet on horses?

The Arts: Design your own jockey silks using paper and watercolors. Create your own outrageous derby hat.

Music: Sing songs that are sung before some of the big races: "Run for the Roses," "My Old Kentucky Home," and "Maryland, My Maryland." Read books or watch movies with horses as a main character (e.g., *Black Beauty* or *National Velvet*, with a young Elizabeth Taylor).

Exercise: Take a trip to a local stable and walk around and look at the horses.

Humor: Have a contest to come up with the wackiest name for a race horse, such as "Too Hot to Handle"!

Old Sayings: "You can lead a horse to water, but you can't make him drink." "Don't look a gift horse in the mouth."

Sensory: Enjoy the vibrant colors and patterns on the jockey silks. Feel and smell the leather saddle.

Early Dementia: Plan a day at the races. Enjoy the food and beautiful horses.

Conversation: Ask a trivia question: "What is labeled as the most exciting two minutes in sports?" (Kentucky Derby) Ask for information: "What is the difference between a trifecta (picking the top three winning horses in order) and an exacta (picking the top two winning horses in order)?" Reminisce: "Maria, did you ride your horse sidesaddle?" Ponder: "James, would you like to be a jockey?" Be curious: "Grayson, I wonder why horses are measured in 'hands' versus 'feet.'"

If the Shoe Fits

Discussing shoes can be a fun way to reminisce about fashion, life events, or travel. *Persons* with dementia, especially both men and women who have a "thing" for shoes, may enjoy this activity.

The Basics

Before Class: Research information on shoes, including fashions, types of shoes, costs of shoes, and purposes of shoes. Gather as many different kinds of shoes as possible, including unusual ones, such as snow shoes, wooden shoes, or combat boots. Visit a vintage clothing store or garage sale for shoes from different time periods. Collect other items related to shoes, such as a shoe horn or shoe tree.

At Class Time: Set the shoes around for everyone to look at. Discuss the different types of shoes and fashions. Invite *persons* to model a favorite pair. Spend time talking about the many kinds of shoes being worn in the room.

Variations: Use an old boot as a planter. Have an ugly shoe contest in which everyone cleans out his or her closet to bring in the ugliest shoe! Take some time to polish a pair of shoes during the activity.

The 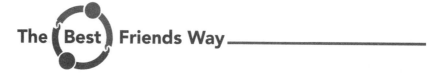 Best Friends Way

Life Story: Does the *person* have a favorite type of shoe to wear? What types of shoes has the *person* worn in his or her lifetime: running shoes, dancing shoes, work boots? Who has difficulty passing up a shoe sale? Did anyone ever work in a shoe store?

The Arts: Using fashion magazines, create a collage about shoes. Decorate old sneakers to give them new life!

Music: Sing "These Boots Are Made for Walking."

Exercise: Take a walk and discuss whether everyone's shoes were good for walking (see Daily Intentional Walking, p. 69).

Humor: Wear a pair of large clown shoes and clown around for the group! Joke about stepping into a puddle and getting your shoes and socks soaked! Joke with the ladies about fashion versus comfort.

Old Sayings: "Walk a mile in my shoes." "Those are big shoes to fill." "He is a shoe-in." "Shoe-shine."

Old Skills: Tying and polishing shoes may be old skills.

Sensory: Smell the leather of the shoes. Feel the snakeskin cowboy boots. Listen to the sound that is made by tap shoes.

Early Dementia: Clean out the closet and sort shoes to either make an inventory or to make a bag for a local charity.

Conversation: Reminisce: "Bob, did you wear steel-toed shoes while you were working?" Tease: "Mary, you have so many shoes; they must fill up your whole house!" Ask for information: "Debbie, did you keep your daughter's first pair of shoes? I've known people who have had them bronzed." Ask for fashion advice: "George, do you think the Italians make the best shoes?"

The Basics ————————————

Before Class: Research Oktoberfest and German culture. Gather items related to Germany and Oktoberfest, such as traditional German clothes, favorite Oktoberfest songs, and beer steins. Prepare traditional Oktoberfest foods, such as sausages, sauerkraut, sauerbraten, Black Forest cake, bunzas (see Making Bunzas, p. 143), and nonalcoholic beer. Download pictures of Germany from the Internet or obtain materials from a travel agent or tourist office. Some of these activities lend themselves well to the Planning Group (p. 163).

At Class Time: Greet the group with a traditional German greeting, "Guten Tag" (see Bonjour or Hola!, p. 29). Pass around the items, and discuss the origins of the celebration. Play festive German music, such as polka tunes or music by brass bands, sample the traditional German foods, and serve nonalcoholic beer in steins, if possible.

Variation: You can also prepare some of the food during class.

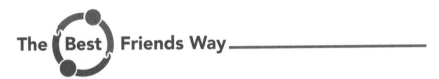

The Best Friends Way ————————————

Life Story: Is the *person* from Germany? Does the *person* have a German heritage? Has the *person* attended an Oktoberfest celebration before? Did he or she enjoy drinking beer? Did he or she ever make sauerkraut?

The Arts: Look up artwork by German artists, including painters and musicians (e.g., Mozart). Find fun photographs or paintings of Oktoberfest activities on the Internet, print them, and pass them around.

Music: Invite an accordion player to entertain.

Exercise: Exercise the arms by swinging your "beer mugs" left to right to the sound of music.

Old Sayings: "German chocolate cake." "German shepherd."

Sensory: The smell of sausage and sauerkraut coupled with the festive sounds of polka music puts everyone in the mood to celebrate!

Early Dementia: Celebrate Oktoberfest with an outing to a German restaurant.

Conversation: Speculate: "Why do we celebrate Oktoberfest in September?" Ask an opinion: "Mark, do you like Black Forest cake?" Seek information: "Gerhardt, did your family celebrate Oktoberfest when you lived in Germany?" Ask for information: "Virginia, tell me about your vacations to Germany. Did you visit Bavaria or the Black Forest?"

Oktoberfest

Oktoberfest is a traditional celebration that involves good food, festive music, and fun. Many *persons* with dementia will recall this festive German holiday and may have been to Oktoberfest celebrations in the United States or in Europe.

Hail to the Chief

United States presidential history can be an interesting subject for many. *Persons* with dementia often have a favorite president, and the ever-changing world of politics provides for lively and meaningful discussion.

The Basics

Before Class: Research information on the presidents. Find a poster/picture of all of the presidents. Collect election memorabilia. Learn if your home state has sent someone to the White House.

At Class Time: Discuss both fun and historical information about the presidents. Examples include the following:

- Only person to hold the two highest offices (president and chief justice): William Howard Taft
- He signed a bill creating the Smithsonian Institution in 1846: James Polk
- He was the youngest president, taking office at the age of 42: Theodore Roosevelt

Discuss the origins of Presidents Day. Ask someone to read the Presidential Oath aloud to the group. Reminisce with the *person* about the presidents of his or her lifetime or leaders *persons* admired.

The 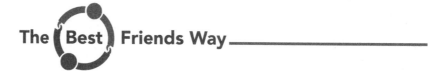 Best Friends Way

Life Story: Has the *person* ever held a political office or run for president of a club or association? Has the *person* or a family member been politically involved? Did someone come from a town with a rich political history (e.g., Chicago)?

The Arts: Look at famous presidential art (e.g., Washington Crossing the Delaware).

Music: Remember the theme songs that were used by some presidents in their campaigns. Listen to patriotic music, such as "Hail to the Chief," "The Star Spangled Banner," or "You're a Grand Old Flag."

Exercise: March or exercise to patriotic music.

Humor: Some political satire may be appropriate and enjoyable. Look at the political cartoons in the newspaper.

Old Skills: Voting and participating in political activities may be an old skill and interest for many.

Early Dementia: Encourage the *person* to remain active in the political process by continuing to vote and becoming an advocate for other *persons* with dementia.

Late Dementia: Many *persons* will recognize political slogans or names and nicknames of presidents from when they were younger.

Conversation: Reminisce: "Olive, do you remember the first time you went to vote?" Ask for information: "Who was the first president to live in the White House?" (John Adams) Debate a general question: "Is it a good thing for young people to be interested in politics?"

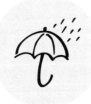

An ounce of prevention . . .

Carefully skip political issues, such as war or current controversies, that could cause dissention.

The Basics

Before Class: Collect information and trivia about spring. Research spring on the Internet using keywords: seasons and springtime. Gather items that are associated with spring, such as spring flowers, fresh fruit, spring hats, pictures of springtime settings, and even items that are related to baseball spring training.

At Class Time: Begin by asking the group what comes to mind when thinking of springtime (e.g., March madness basketball tournaments, bird nesting, longer days, receding snow, green grass). Write these ideas on a flipchart and discuss these with the group. Enjoy fresh springtime fruit while looking at the springtime items. Sing a song about springtime or model spring hats. Bring in a litter of kittens or puppies to symbolize the bounty of spring.

Spring Has Sprung

Springtime is a time of renewal and happiness for many people, with opportunities to venture outside after a winter of being cooped up inside (at least in many parts of the world). This activity invites *persons* with dementia to celebrate and reminisce about spring.

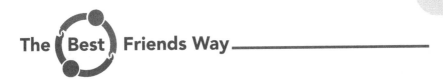

The (Best) Friends Way

Life Story: What is the *person's* favorite season? What activities did the *person* do in the spring? What was spring like where *persons* grew up? Who has seen the cherry trees bloom in Washington, D.C.? Did anyone plant spring bulbs?

The Arts: Create a springtime-themed bulletin board (see A Tree for All Seasons, p. 138). Write a poem about spring. Make May baskets. Arrange fresh flowers.

Exercise: Take a walk in the springtime air. Dance around a may pole (see Group Dancing, p. 75)

Humor: Laugh about the old saying, "In the spring a young man's fancy lightly turns to thoughts of love."

Old Sayings: "April showers bring May flowers." "Spring is in the air." "Merry month of May." "Spring forward."

Old Skills: Encourage your group to help you with spring cleaning.

Sensory: Take a walk outside and listen for all of the springtime sounds: a gentle breeze, birds chirping, lawn mowers out for the first mow of the season. Enjoy the smell and sensations of a fresh spring shower.

Spirituality: Springtime is the season for the renewal of life. Explore Easter and other festivals of the rites of spring.

Early Dementia: Ask the *person* to read aloud a poem about spring.

Late Dementia: Aromas can evoke the sensations of spring (see Stop and Smell the Roses, p. 76).

Conversation: Speculate: "I wonder why we do only spring cleaning. Why not fall or summer cleaning?" Ask for information: "Josephine, why do we spring forward with our clocks?" Talk to someone about farm life: "Isn't spring the time of birthing for all of the farm animals?"

Autumn Leaves

Autumn brings back many memories for most people, such as going back to school, harvest, and football. *Persons* with dementia may enjoy discussing the season of autumn and participating in traditional autumn activities.

The Basics

Before Class: Collect information and trivia about the seasons and autumn. Research these topics on the Internet using keywords: seasons, autumn, harvest, Labor Day, and Thanksgiving.

Gather items that are associated with autumn, such as fall vegetables, farming equipment for harvesting, a football, fall leaves, and pictures of autumn settings. Decorate the room with fall vegetables and beautifully colored leaves. Prepare apple fritters or apple cider (see Planning Group, p. 163).

At Class Time: Pass out apple fritters and cider to spark memories of autumn. Discuss some of the group's favorite activities and memories of autumn (e.g., hayrides, hiking, bonfires, football). Pass around autumn items to look at and spark discussion. Make the most of fall holidays, such as Halloween and Thanksgiving.

The (Best) Friends Way

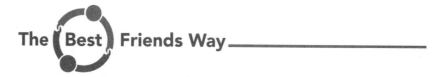

Life Story: What was the *person's* favorite season? Was the *person* an avid football fan? Did the *person* grow up on a farm where they harvested in autumn? What was autumn like where they grew up? Did he or she make a tradition of going to New England to look at the changing leaves each year? Did he or she have any special way of making Thanksgiving turkey and stuffing?

The Arts: Use the leaves that decorate the room to create leaf prints (see Rubbings, p. 130).

Music: Sing together "Shine on, Harvest Moon."

Exercise: Enjoy the crisp fall air by taking a walk to look at the changing leaves. Gather some fallen leaves for decorating.

Humor: Laugh about jumping into a large pile of leaves just after someone finished raking them!

Old Sayings: "Fall back." "October's bright blue weather."

Old Skills: Memories of canning may spark the *person* to practice the old skill.

Sensory: Enjoy the sweet aroma and taste of warm apple cider. Feel the texture of the different types of leaves that you have collected.

Spirituality: Discuss the cycles of growth and harvest, which are symbolic of life.

Early Dementia: Take a drive to go "leaf peeping."

Conversation: Reminisce: "Did you enjoy raking leaves in the fall?" Recall the life story: "Jim, you always enjoyed tailgating and football games every fall." Be mischievous: "Should we liven things up by putting a little rum in the cider?" Celebrate the life story: "Hazel, where did you learn to can vegetables?"

The Basics

Before Class: Collect information and trivia about Mexico, including history and popular tourist attractions. Research Mexico using Internet keywords: Mexico and Mayan Ruins. Gather items from Mexico, including pieces of art, pictures of Mexico taken from tourist brochures or the Internet, a poncho or other traditional costumes, inexpensive pottery from a garden store, or other ideas. Hang a map of Mexico with colorful thumbtacks highlighting the places that you plan to "visit" during class time. Prepare a traditional Mexican food, such as huevos rancheros or Mexican hot chocolate (traditionally flavored with cinnamon).

At Class Time: Pass around the items from Mexico and discuss them. Share Mexican history and trivia, including information about the Mayan or other ancient peoples. List major Mexican cities and chart them on a map. Discuss the Mexican culture (e.g., traditions, holidays). Discuss the importance of the siesta. Taste the food and take a poll on who likes Mexican food and who does not.

Tip: Invite staff members who have lived in Mexico to share their experiences.

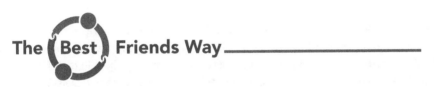

The (Best) Friends Way

Life Story: Did anyone ever live in Mexico? Has anyone traveled to Mexico? Is anyone of Mexican descent? Who speaks Spanish? Has anyone enjoyed making or eating corn husk–wrapped tamales?

The Arts: Enjoy a painting by Diego Rivera, a famous Mexican artist. Paint pots using colorful Mexican designs.

Music: Invite a mariachi band to entertain your group or listen to some upbeat, vibrant Mexican music on the radio.

Exercise: Encourage the group members to join you in a Mexican hat dance.

Humor: Debate whether it is better to stay at a beach resort or visit museums and cultural sites.

Old Skills: Some individuals may enjoy studying maps.

Sensory: Enjoy the taste and aroma of the food.

Spirituality: Explore some of Mexico's spiritual rituals and traditions, such as the Shrine of Guadalupe or the Day of the Dead.

Late Dementia: Share a taste of the Mexican version of hot chocolate (has a cinnamon taste and is a bit spicy).

Conversation: Reminisce: "Fred, you honeymooned in the Riviera Maya, right?" Start a friendly debate about the benefits of travel: "Madge, do you like to travel or would you rather stay home?" Share some dreams: "Where would you like to travel if you could go to just one place?" Tease: "Mike, is it true that you like your food very hot and spicy?"

Touring Mexico

Traveling has been a pastime for many *persons*, and Mexico remains a popular tourist destination. *Persons* with dementia may enjoy talking about visiting Mexico in this activity that involves a fantasy tour of Mexico.

An ounce of prevention . . .

Go easy on the often hot spices associated with Mexican cuisine!

101

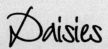

Daisies

Flowers have universal appeal because of their beauty, fragrance, and history. *Persons* with dementia often maintain an interest in flowers, and this activity involving daisies can serve as a template for almost any flower.

The Basics

Choose a flower that is native to your area or season. For the purpose of this activity, we have chosen the daisy.

Before Class: Collect information and trivia about daisies; for example, a purple species that is native to the lower Mississippi basin is called a Western daisy. Research daisies on the Internet using the keyword *daisy*. Gather daisies from a local gardener or florist to display during class time. Choose a variety of colors and sizes.

At Class Time: Discuss information and trivia about daisies. Discuss the various types, such as the Gerber, Shasta, and African daisy, and let each *person* choose his or her favorite one.

Variation: Bring in small pots, potting soil, and daisy plants. Plant some daisies, then check their growth each day.

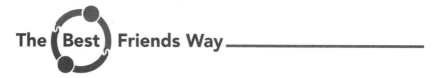

The (Best) Friends Way

Life Story: Did anyone grow daisies? Who in the group had a "green thumb" and was an excellent gardener (or not)? Does anyone have some special memories of daisies, perhaps gathering wild daisies as a child or having them in their family home? Has anyone had a family member, close friend, or dog named Daisy?

The Arts: Create a flower arrangement using different colors of daisies. Make a lei from daisies. Put together an art project involving drawings, collages, or other images of flowers.

Music: Sing the song "Daisy, Daisy, give me your answer do. . . ."

Exercise: Take a walk through a garden and admire daisies together.

Humor: Humorously play the childhood game of "He Loves Me, He Loves Me Not," in which you pull off the petals of a daisy one at a time until the final petal determines whether "he" loves you.

Old Sayings: "Daisy chain." "Fresh as a daisy."

Old Skills: Gardening and planting flowers are old skills for many *persons*.

Sensory: Enjoy the variety of bright colors and patterns in the daisies.

Early Dementia: Always be aware of good readers who love to share this skill. Let them read some of the trivia about daisies.

Late Dementia: The daisy is such a familiar flower. *Persons* may enjoy seeing a daisy or touching it.

Conversation: Ask an opinion: "Which color daisy do you like best?" Reminisce: "Judy, your wedding bouquet was made of daisies, right?" Ask for information: "What is a Shasta daisy?" Reminisce: "Harold, did you have wild daisies growing on your farm in New Hampshire?"

The Basics ———————————

Before Class: Research the history of "keeping cool." Gather various kinds of fans to look at and discuss. Handheld examples include decorative folding fans from Japan or other cultures, Chinese sandalwood fans that have a beautiful fragrance, cardboard fans from churches or funeral homes, and battery-operated handheld fans. Research how fans are used to convey a message (e.g., fan dancing, flirting).

At Class Time: Look at fans together and discuss each one. Discuss whether the room is too hot or too cold. Create an art project to make and/or decorate fans. Share some history or trivia about the use of fans.

Variation: Write the word *FAN* at the top of a flipchart. Ask the group to change the letter F to another letter that makes a new word, such as "can," "Dan," "ban," "man," and see how many words can be created.

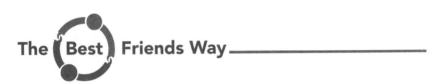

The (Best) Friends Way ———————————

Life Story: Did the *person* have a collection of fans or use a fan as a young girl? Did the *person* grow up in a warm climate or in a cooler climate, where fans might not have been used? Did the *person* grow up with a window fan to cool the bedroom? Who has had a ceiling or an attic fan?

The Arts: Study the artwork on fans from various cultures. Make colorful fans from tie-dyed tissue paper (see Volume One, Creating Wrapping Paper, p. 80).

Exercise: Fanning each other can be great exercise for your arms.

Humor: Tease the men in the room about whether they have ever used a fan. Take today's newspaper and make an oversized fan with it! There are also dozens of "how hot is it?" jokes on the Internet: "How hot is it? It was so hot that you could fry an egg on the sidewalk!"

Sensory: Enjoy the intricate designs on the decorative folding fans. Experience the feeling of the breeze on your skin.

Late Dementia: *Persons* may enjoy the cool breeze of being fanned.

Conversation: Reminisce: "Do you remember when we didn't have air conditioning? How did you keep cool then?" Explore information: "Gretchen, did you know that the way you hold a fan can carry a message?" Reminisce: "Can you remember the hottest place you've ever lived?" Check an attitude: "Do you like hot or cold weather?"

Handheld Fans

Handheld fans are used in every culture—sometimes to make individuals more comfortable on a hot day or in a hot room, other times to communicate a message. Fans offer wonderful opportunities to interact, reminisce, and have fun. *Persons* with dementia can take the opportunity to teach the younger generation about fans.

Astrology

Individuals who believe in astrology look at particular personality traits and compare them with traits that are associated with the placement of the planets in the sky when a *person* was born. *Persons* with dementia enjoy the opportunity to give their own opinion about astrology: whether they are believers, are skeptics, or simply enjoy this as a fun pastime.

The Basics

Before Class: Gather name tags, lists of sun signs (Aries, Taurus, Gemini, Cancer, Leo, Virgo, Libra, Scorpio, Sagittarius, Capricorn, Aquarius, and Pisces), pictures of the symbols of sun signs, and lists of participant birthdays. Create a brief description of each sign (a few sentences is enough). Write everyone's preferred name on the name tag, followed by the month and day of his or her birth.

Some good Web sites to visit are www.astrology-numerology.com and www.astrology-online.com.

At Class Time: Read each astrological description and talk about the qualities of each sign. Go around the group, identify each person's birth date, and announce his or her astrological sign. Read the positive attributes of individuals with that sign.

Variations: Look at the horoscopes in the newspaper every morning and read aloud any upbeat or humorous advice. Also, list famous people and their signs (e.g., Ronald Reagan, Aquarius).

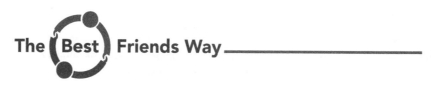 The **Best** Friends Way

Life Story: Has astrology been an interest of the *person* in the past? Has anyone ever had his or her fortune told? Tie the person's daily horoscope to something from his or her personality or life story (e.g., "Today's horoscope discusses wisdom. Professor Clark, you've always been a very wise man!").

Music: "Aquarius" by the Fifth Dimension.

Humor: "The moon affects the tide, and the untied." [An old saying about the full moon impacting nature as well as romance!]

Spirituality: The spiritual idea of being a part of a greater universe connects us with the human species in all times and places.

Early Dementia: Ask a *person* to help by reading one of the lists. The *person* may enjoy going a little deeper into astrology by adding a component, such as moon signs (the position of the moon when you were born affects the emotions, according to some astrologers) or numerology (the study of numbers).

Late Dementia: Gently validate the *person's* finer qualities.

Conversation: Laugh and joke: "Georgia, I know what your sign is; you must be a Virgo to pay such wonderful attention to the details of the work you do." Find something in common: "You and I are both Aquarians. We want to save the world!" Speculate on the meaning of life: "Buzz, what else do you think we can learn from the stars?" Seek information: "Nawanta, do you know anyone who has ever been to an astrologer for advice?"

An ounce of prevention . . .

Some individuals may feel uncomfortable with astrology because of religious beliefs or life attitudes. Keep the atmosphere light, rather than serious, and allow a person to participate at any level that he or she wishes.

The Basics ⎯⎯⎯⎯⎯⎯⎯⎯⎯

Before Class: Gather Halloween trivia and facts from the Internet. Get materials for simple costumes. Shop for Halloween candy and decorations. Get ingredients for baking cookies or other treats.

At Class Time: Following are some suggestions to make Halloween fun and successful for *persons* with dementia:

- Make decorations: Any artwork done in Halloween colors (orange, black, yellow, and purple) will send the message that it is time to have fun. Make simple costumes.
- Hold a contest: Halloween is a great time for a hat contest. Hats can be decorated, put on and taken off easily, and make a big difference. Everyone can wear a hat, and everyone can vote on which one they find the most creative or silliest.
- Decorate pumpkins (see Decorating Pumpkins, p. 180).
- Encourage staff members to dress up.
- Decorate cookies with Halloween themes, and serve other party foods.

Variation: Invite a class of schoolchildren to come and trick or treat for the program and hand out candy and cookies to them as their reward.

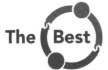

The (Best) Friends Way ⎯⎯⎯⎯⎯⎯⎯⎯

Life Story: Does the *person* have any particular interest in or aversion to Halloween? Has the *person* celebrated Halloween during different life stages: in childhood, early adulthood, or now? If so, then how? Did anyone grow up in a country where Halloween was not well known?

Humor: Vote on which staff member has the funniest costume!

Sensory: Bright colors of the decorations and costumes light up the visual senses. Often the materials that are used to make costumes are more sensory than usual clothes. Touch and enjoy!

Spirituality: Enjoy the spirit of giving and of enjoying children.

Early Dementia: Enlist the *person's* help in planning how the costumes should be judged.

Late Dementia: Celebrate the sights, sounds, and aromas.

Conversation: Ask a question from long-term memory: "Mari, what did you think of Halloween when you first came here from Peru?" Reminisce: "Did you ever make popcorn balls to give to the children on Halloween?" Make a funny suggestion: "Antoine, did you ever pull any tricks on Halloween?"

Halloween

Halloween has become one of America's favorite times for decorating, partying, and fun. *Persons* with dementia also enjoy coming up with new ideas and stretching the limits a bit, or just observing the comings and goings of young people who are excited about the holiday.

An ounce of prevention . . .

Persons with dementia can have perception problems and may misunderstand anything that is too seriously ghoulish. Avoid foods that are created to look like eyeballs, witches' fingers, and other scary things. Some people might not want to celebrate Halloween because of religious preferences.

Horsing Around

Horses have been linked to the human race since the beginning of recorded history. *Persons* with dementia have had various opportunities to relate to horses and many may be passionate about this other "best friend."

The Basics

Before Class: Go on the Internet and search for facts about the horse: the origin, different breeds, ancient drawings of horses, and the Pony Express. Gather picture books of different breeds of horses. Find items related to horses, such as horseshoes, saddle, bridle, riding cap, and boots.

- Flipchart and markers

At Class Time: Use cards to record facts that were collected about horses. Present some of these facts, such as where the horse was thought to have originated, information about ancient drawings of horses, the history of the Pony Express, and some common breeds of horses. Pass around and discuss the items related to horses. Encourage *persons* to talk about experiences they have had with horses. Using the flipchart, ask *persons* to recall as many ways as possible that horses have been used through the centuries. Play a game of horse trivia.

Variations: Bring a horse or miniature pony to the program for all to enjoy. Visit a horse farm. Also, see A Day at the Races, p. 95, for more ideas.

The (Best) Friends Way

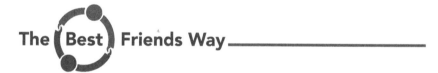

Life Story: Mine the life story for clues to *persons'* interest in horses, such as showing ponies or horses in competition, cultivating the fields with horses, selling equipment for horses, raising and caring for horses, or riding for fun. Did anyone have a pony to ride? Did anyone play the ponies at the track?

The Arts: Make a guide with simple lines for drawing a horse; encourage *persons* to try to draw a horse. Show some ancient drawings of horses. Talk about the book *Black Beauty*.

Music: Choose one of the following to sing: "Over the river and through the woods to grandmother's house we go," "Put on your old gray bonnet," "Love and marriage go together like a horse and carriage."

Exercise: Play a game of horseshoes using lightweight, indoor horseshoes.

Old Sayings: "You can lead a horse to water, but you can't make him drink." "That is a horse of a different color." "Hold your horses!"

Sensory: Encourage *persons* to feel the leather of the saddle and experience the weight of the horseshoe.

Conversation: Reminisce: "Dicy, did you ever ride a wooden horse on a merry-go-round?" Ask a question: "Salvador, which way do you hang this horseshoe for good luck? Do you hang the curved part turned up or down?" Share a story: "Bessie, I had a stick horse when I was a child. It was made out of a broomstick. Did you ever ride a stick horse?"

The Basics

Before Class: Brainstorm all of the ways in which the number 5 can be used in all of the segments of a 4-hour program, such as in decorating, preparing snacks, being together during informal and reminiscing times, exercising, playing games, and enjoying special projects.

At Class Time: Incorporate the number 5 in all aspects of your program.

Adapted from Field of Themes: 100 Activities for Our Senior Friends *(2006) by Barbara Fister, RN, MA, Director, and Sylvia "Skippy" Valentine, LMSW, Volunteer Team Leader of My Friend's Place, Bangor, ME (see Appendix 2).*

Variation: This program can be shortened for a brief activity or expanded for a day-long or even week-long activity.

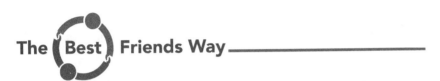

The (Best) Friends Way

Life Story: Who in the group has five children, worked 5 days a week, got up at 5 o'clock, has five grandchildren, was born in May (the fifth month), or has five sisters? Does anyone wear a size 5 shoe? Who had to practice the "five-finger exercise" when taking piano lessons? Has anyone ever met a five-star general? Does anyone consider the number 5 to be his or her lucky number?

The Arts: Decorate with items in groups of five, such as five vases, five stuffed gloves standing in a row, or five easels waiting for five artists to go to work.

Music: Sing "Five Foot Two, Eyes of Blue."

Exercise: Clap hands five times above the head, behind the back, to the right, to the left, and to the front. Repeat. Give the *person* to the right a "high five" and repeat with the *person* on the left. Using five softballs and five containers lined up in a row, encourage *persons* to try to toss one ball in each container.

Old Sayings: "Fifth wheel." "High five." "5 o'clock shadow." "The fabulous five." "The five senses." "Counting by fives." "The Jackson 5."

Sensory: Make smoothies using five ingredients: bananas, strawberries, yogurt, orange juice, and milk. Enjoy the textures of the fruits and taste of the smoothie.

Early Dementia: Research numerology; have *persons* read statements about the meaning of the number 5.

Conversation: Laugh together: "Sadie, the kids give me a high five all the time. Do you think we are too old for this silly stuff?" Reminisce: "Rachael, did you ever buy a 5-cent ice cream cone?" Ask for help: "Norman, help me think of all of the words that rhyme with five." Debate with a mechanic: "Mike, there are four-cylinder and six-cylinder cars. Are there five-cylinder cars?"

Hanukkah: The Festival of Lights

Hanukkah is celebrated on the twenty-fifth day of the Jewish calendar month of Kislev and lasts for 8 days and 8 nights. It celebrates the triumphs—both religious and military—of ancient Jewish heroes. It usually falls somewhere in the month of December. Though it is a minor holiday, it has rich symbolic value to Jewish families. *Persons* with dementia can enjoy the celebratory spirit and meaning of Hanukkah.

The Basics

Before Class: Go on the Internet, consult books and pamphlets, and/or arrange to have a member of the Jewish community come to your program and discuss the meaning of Hanukkah. Bring in a menorah (a candle stand with nine branches). Obtain a dreidel (a traditional spinning top used in a child's game).

At Class Time: Share the information you have learned about Hanukkah, including history and fun facts. Pass around the menorah and explain how a candle is lit for each of the 8 nights using the tall candle in the middle. Play a game with the dreidel. Invite any Jewish participants to share childhood memories of Hanukkah, or share memories of their children's or grandchildren's experiences.

Traditional foods, such as latkes, potato pancakes, can be fried and served with apple sauce and sour cream.

At the close of each class, invite someone to light the candle for that day and share a traditional blessing (see also Judaism, p. 63).

Submitted by Julie Lamberti, LCSW, Director, House of Welcome Adult Day Services of the North Shore Senior Center, Northfield, IL.

The (Best) Friends Way

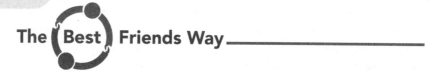

Life Story: Note who in the group is Jewish and may celebrate this and other Jewish holidays. If he or she has children or grandchildren, then encourage their attendance at the class. Can anyone in the group teach others a few words of Hebrew? Did anyone celebrate Hanukkah in Israel?

The Arts: Using almost any art form, participants can make paintings or representations of the symbols of Hanukkah: dreidel, menorah, candles.

Music: Play traditional music during your class or during the 8 days of Hanukkah to experience the joy of the holiday.

Old Sayings: Hanukkah gelt (gifts of real or chocolate coins given to children during the holiday).

Sensory: Enjoy the traditional sweets and other foods during this time of year.

Spirituality: Discuss other Jewish traditions and holidays with the group. Ask a Jewish youth group to come in and sing and/or visit with the residents.

Conversation: Recall vivid memories: "Mr. Zeff, can you tell us about how you celebrated Hanukkah with your children?" Compare: "Madge, you've lived in Israel and in the United States; is there a big difference in how Hanukkah is celebrated in the two countries?" Start something fun: "Harry, show everyone how you spin the dreidel!"

The Basics

Before Class: Gather information and trivia about maple syrup harvesting, production, and products, including pictures of gathering maple sap from a bucket hanging on a tree, Native American traditions, what maple sugar actually is, and "sugar shacks" (huts used to process the syrup).

- Purchase maple syrup, candies, or cookies

At Class Time: Use your creativity to devise an entertaining class. Share trivia and facts about the maple harvest that you have learned from the Internet. Show off a Canadian flag with the maple-leaf motif. Create a Maple Harvest festival at your site that can involve baking, tasting, walks outside, a pancake breakfast, and games and contests.

Variation: Make a bulletin board celebrating the theme.

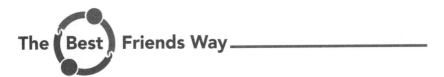

The Best Friends Way

Life Story: Did anyone grow up in New England, eastern Canada, or another region that is known for its maple syrup production? Who likes pancakes with maple syrup? Is anyone proud of his or her French Canadian background?

The Arts: Create a maple tree bulletin board or spring harvest poster. Bake maple-flavored treats. Use maple leaves to make leaf prints (see Rubbings, p. 130).

Exercise: Spring can be a time to encourage all to spend more time out-of-doors and look for maple trees.

Sensory: Taste the very sweet maple flavor in syrups, cookies, or candies. Feel the syrup's stickiness. Make some pancakes!

Early Dementia: Take a field trip to a festival, farm, or pancake house!

Late Dementia: Enjoy the taste of maple candy.

Music: Sing "O Canada," the national anthem of Canada.

Conversation: Discuss a favorite trip: "Eve, have you been to eastern Canada or New England?" Vote: "Do you like chocolate or maple flavor better?" Taste together: "Let's have a bit of maple candy to celebrate springtime!" Enjoy each other: "Mike, did you get enough pancakes at the famous restaurant that I told you about?" Ponder: "Alex, do all maple trees produce sap?"

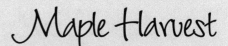

Maple Harvest

Late winter and early spring are traditionally the time of year to harvest sap from maple trees.

Northern Lights

Few of us have witnessed, but many of us have been fascinated by, the northern lights (Aurora Borealis). *Persons* with dementia will enjoy participating in a program on this spectacular natural phenomenon.

The Basics

Before Class: Research information on the northern lights, such as the history, science, and folklore. Acquire pictures or a video of the northern lights.

At Class Time: Pass the pictures around for the group to enjoy and discuss. Post a map in the room to point out locations where the northern lights can be seen. Share history and folklore to spark discussion. A good Internet site is www.northern-lights.no/.

Some fun facts include the following: The northern lights first gained attention through Galileo, the famed 16th-century astronomer, but a Norwegian chronicle from approximately 1230 AD mentions them. In Latin, *aurora borealis* means "flame of red." They have been described as a "heavenly ballet." They primarily appear in winter in the Northern Hemisphere.

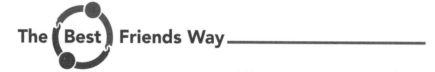

The (Best) Friends Way

Life Story: Has anyone traveled to see the northern lights? Is anyone from the regions where northern lights can be seen? Does anyone come from a Native American or Nordic background, in which the lights are revered? Is anyone an artist who would appreciate the dramatic lights and colors? Has anyone ever witnessed this display of color?

The Arts: Marvel at photographs of the northern lights. Create a watercolor painting (see Watercolor Techniques, p. 134) in the spirit of the northern lights or any art project that celebrates color.

Music: While talking about the lights, put on some gentle classical music to set the tone.

Humor: Joke about whether it would be worth it to go outside on a very cold night to see the lights or you should skip them and stay inside, where it's warm.

Sensory: Try a simple visualization exercise: Ask all present to close their eyes and try to visualize the lights.

Spirituality: The lights have great spiritual meaning to Native Americans, who see God reflected in Nature.

Early Dementia: Involve the *person* in research about the topic. For example, are the northern lights the same colors as a rainbow?

Conversation: Make a life story connection: "Lars, can you remember when you first saw the lights growing up in Denmark?" "Paul, did your parents talk to you about the lights when you were growing up in Alaska?" Evoke a dream: "How many of you would like to see the lights if you have not already?" Ask anyone who has seen the lights to share their memories.

The Basics ━━━━━━━━━━━━━

Before Class: Obtain an oversized picture of the Mona Lisa through the Internet, a company that sells posters such as www.art.com, or by purchasing an oversized art book (the Mona Lisa appears in many books, including ones often on a discount shelf at bookstores). Go on the Internet to gather information about the painting and about its creator, Leonardo da Vinci.

At Class Time: Display the image in a small-group environment. Share information and trivia about da Vinci and the painting from the Internet and discuss this famous work of art.

Ask some easy questions, such as:

- Have you ever been to Paris, France? (Many *persons* with dementia will recall this because travel to Paris is such a vivid memory. Cross-reference with life stories if possible.)
- Do you think the Mona Lisa is beautiful?
- Why do you think the Mona Lisa is smiling?
- [Holding the painting] Can you see how her eyes seem to follow us as we look at her from different angles? [Comment on the mastery of da Vinci's technique and skills.]

Allow time for reminiscence and discussion. Play Nat King Cole's famed song "Mona Lisa" to end the program.

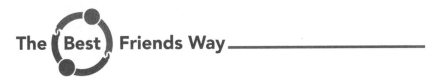

The (Best) Friends Way ━━━━━━━━━━

Life Story: Has anyone been to the Louvre or any other famous art museum? Is anyone of French descent? Ask the ladies whether they ever enjoyed French perfume.

The Arts: Make a collage of pictures of people with interesting smiles or collect pictures of animals that seem to be smiling. Encourage the group to do some freestyle drawings of their interpretation of the Mona Lisa.

Exercise: Visit a local art museum (see Partnering with a Museum, p. 209).

Humor: Ask the group whether Mona needs a "makeover," with a new hairdo and jewelry.

Sensory: Try a guided relaxation tour to Paris, France (see Guided Relaxation, p. 80).

Early Dementia: Ask a *person* to help plan the activity and to read some of the historic facts about the painting.

Late Dementia: *Persons* may enjoy the song "Mona Lisa."

Conversation: Ask an opinion: "Simon, do you think Mona Lisa looks happy?" or "Do you think that her hairdo is becoming?" Ponder: "Coach, what do you think Mona Lisa is smiling about?" Laugh together: "Paul, do you think she would be fun on a date?" Ask for advice: "Garnett, what would you do to help Mona Lisa improve her wardrobe?"

Mona Lisa

The Mona Lisa is arguably the most famous painting in the world. Use it to create a fun classroom activity or small-group activity. *Persons* with dementia will enjoy learning about the painting, reminiscing about a trip to Paris if they have been, and discussing the mysteries of the masterpiece by Leonardo da Vinci.

CHAPTER SEVEN

Let's Create

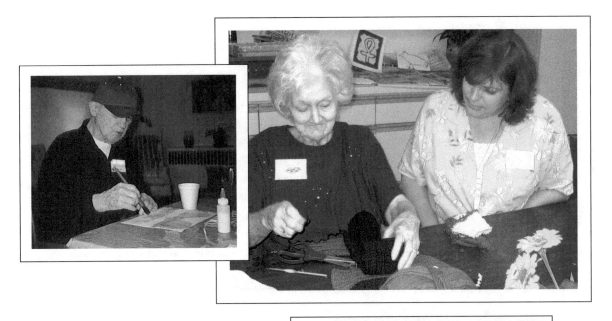

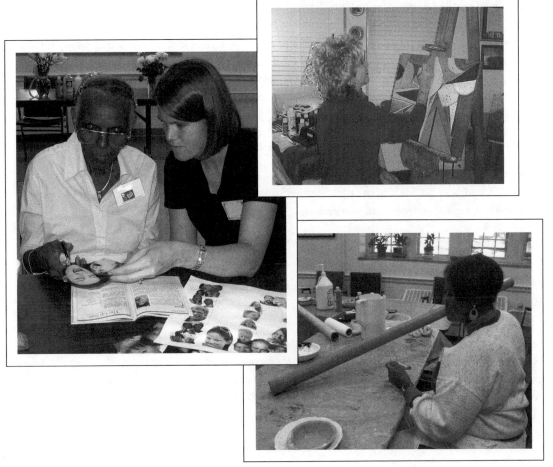

Let's Create

In speaking to activities professionals around the United States, it seems as though there are two camps when it comes to creative arts activities. Some activities staff thrive on creative arts projects and have a natural interest and talent in this area. They could have their own television show on the Home and Garden Network! Others are less experienced in this arena or lack confidence to jump in. The activities in this chapter will appeal to both of these camps—the experienced staff "crafter" as well as the newcomer.

The goals of the activities in this chapter are to increase self-esteem, to provide a sense of belonging through socialization, to provide a new avenue for communication, to provide opportunities for *persons* to have control and make choices, and to increase positive feelings that are associated with making a contribution. Creative arts experiences can be offered through visual art media, music, writing, and creative movement.

As Daphne Gormley, a *person* with early dementia, shared in Chapter 1, "One of the benefits of my art is that it provides me a way of communicating without words." Another reason that art works well even with *persons* who may never have picked up a paintbrush or glue stick in their life is that dementia may actually free up or increase creativity (at least early in the disease). A lawyer who no longer recalls constitutional law may take pleasure in sketching a lovely object. If staff encourage him, then he may produce a drawing of which he is very proud.

We draw your attention to a few specific activities in this chapter:

A Tree for All Seasons (p. 138) is a great group project that can be a focal point for your dementia care unit.

A number of activities involve hands-on work with paints, including Partner Prints (p. 129), Painting with String (p. 135), and Sponge Painting (p. 136). Staff will take delight in learning some of these techniques. They also make for great intergenerational activities.

We like collages because everyone can participate at some level. Blue Collage (p. 120) is easily adapted to other colors.

Many of the projects can be done as a class or group or one-to-one.

Art supplies that are used for visual art projects should be simple, safe, easy to use, and easy to clean. Most art supplies come in nontoxic varieties. Basic supplies to have on hand for visual art projects include paint, paper, a pair of scissors, paintbrushes of many sizes, washable markers, newspapers or plastic tablecloths to cover tables, jars to hold water, white glue, pencils, pens, a ruler, and paper towels. Tempera paints are good to use for most painting experiences. One type of paint that has been found to work especially well for painting projects is BioColor paint from Discount School Supply (www.discountschoolsupply.com). It is used with little mess or waste in twist-top "Nancy" bottles. Most *persons* will have success with cake watercolors as well. Scholastic-grade acrylic paint may also be used if it is nontoxic.

Have lots of paper on hand. Some of the paper must be strong enough to hold paint (50- to 80-lb. weight). Thin paper, such as copier paper, may be used for other projects. For sculptures, use clay that is air-drying, nontoxic, warm, and easy to mold.

The supplies that you have on hand can give you ideas. Many programs receive an abundance of donated magazines. You can also obtain free or low-cost art supplies from lumberyards (scraps, chips), newspaper printing plants (free newsprint), paint supply stores (discontinued wallpaper books), frame shops (unused mats/pieces), marble/monument companies (marble and granite chips), and fabric shops (fabric and felt odds and ends, remnants).

Theme collages may be made with magazines, school glue, construction paper, a pair of scissors, and a little imagination. You may have other unusual items that people have donated, such as old greeting cards, buttons, or yarn. Create special projects using whatever supplies you have. Most small, lightweight items can be used as part of a collage (see list of collage materials on p. 225). Enjoy the creative process by following some of these Best Friends creative activities. Pick a simple activity from the chapter and do it in a 30-minute staff in-service session. Encourage staff members to take home the finished product as a gift for a family member.

Tips for Staff Training: Create a collage around a training issue, such as workplace safety or ways we can thank and recognize each other. Staff members often enjoy something different, and you can make the connection between this activity and a similar activitiy for *persons*.

CHAPTER SEVEN ACTIVITIES

The Basics

Save a number of paintings or art projects as a resource from which to draw for this activity. They can be unfinished paintings, drawings, or basically any kind of artwork that can be redone to make a different project. The possibilities are limitless, and the type of pieces found will dictate the type of "new" artwork that is going to be made.

To start, lay out the old artwork and creatively disassemble the pieces or cut out your favorite part to reuse. Tell the group that famous painters such as Picasso often recycled their own art to come up with new ideas and to save money on art supplies. Either paint over old paintings and add new details or embellishments, or take the pieces and make a collage on a new sheet of paper or "canvas."

Variation: Use recycled art for gift wrapping or for decoupage (see Decoupage Eggs, p. 125).

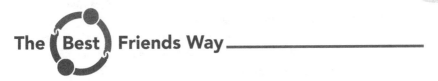

The (Best) Friends Way

Life Story: Was the *person* thrifty? Was the *person* a recycler? Did he or she have an adventurous spirit, willing to try something new?

Old Sayings: "Waste not, want not." "Making something out of nothing."

Old Skills: Cutting, painting, and outlining all are old skills from our early days.

Sensory: Include a variety of materials, colors, and textures.

Spirituality: One of the most beautiful spiritual practices is to live the values that you hold. If you value recycling, then apply the practice to all areas that you can.

Late Dementia: Just being a part of the group and looking at the pieces is a social and sensory experience.

Conversation: Laugh together: "Gilbert, this is our opportunity to create a masterpiece." Ponder: "Maya, what do you think we can do to give this painting a new look?" Acknowledge a common bond: "Tobin, we have two left hands instead of two left feet." Be an art critic with the group: "Do you think Picasso would approve of this? It is our own version of abstract, modern art!"

Recycled Art

Many of us were raised to use everything that we could, to generate little garbage, and to recycle. Today this value is still strong and popular. A *person* with dementia can take pride in the concept of taking something that is not being used and putting it to good use, as in this project in which you make new art from old art.

An ounce of prevention . . .

Some persons may not want to cut up or deface artwork. Others may be upset if their piece is recycled. Use sensitivity and common sense to minimize these problems.

Stained Glass Windows

A stained glass window can be a "never-to-forget" memory. Many *persons* with dementia have marveled at the beautiful stained glass windows in the United States and in other countries. This activity allows them to create their own.

The Basics

- Different colors of cellophane paper
- Two sheets of black construction paper, 8½" × 11" or larger
- Scissors
- Glue
- Ruler

Search the Internet for facts about the history and art of stained glass. When possible, obtain a sample of stained glass art and books on the famous stained glass windows from around the world. Discuss the process of making stained glass and spend time looking through the books. Examine the sample art piece and note the lead that frames the design.

Draw a 1-inch margin all the way around a sheet of black construction paper and cut out the middle. Put aside until the end. This will be the picture frame for your final product.

Draw a 1-inch margin all the way around the second sheet of black construction paper, but do not cut!

Draw a design on the second sheet within the margins. Experiment with the design. It can be very simple—circles, flowers, abstract objects—or a religious theme.

Before cutting out the design, expand the outlines of the pattern a quarter inch to form the frame for the cellophane and to give a dramatic look, much like the lead in real stained glass windows. Cut out the design and all the extra space, leaving the quarter-inch frame around your design.

Cut out pieces of cellophane to fill the empty space. Use different colors. Don't worry if the colors overlap. Glue the cellophane to the back of the design. When completed, glue the whole second page to the back of the first sheet.

Variation: Use colored tissue paper instead of cellophane. Tissue paper comes in a broken-glass motif of many colors in one sheet. This makes the process very easy because it can be glued in one piece to the back of the black construction paper design, letting many colors shine through the window.

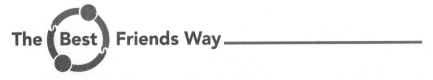

Life Story: Reminisce about someone's trip to Europe, where he or she visited many beautiful cathedrals with elaborate stained glass windows. Find out whether anyone lived in a Victorian house with a stained glass door or window. Suggest designs for the project that relate to the *person's* life.

The Arts: Display the completed window where the sun can shine through for all to enjoy.

Sensory: When the light shines through the colorful paper, it makes a big impression.

Spirituality: Religious symbols can be used as designs.

Early Dementia: Several *persons* could be invited to help prepare the designs for the windows before the class session (see Planning Group, p. 163).

Conversation: Encourage conversation: "Violet, did your church, St. Raphael, have stained glass windows?" Marvel: "Just look at this. It is so beautiful when the sun shines through what we have made." Ask for information: "George, did you ever put stained glass windows in a house or church that you were building?"

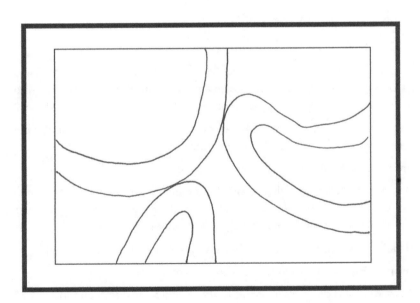

Blue Collage

We all enjoy color for the interest that it provides in our life and the way colors make us feel. *Persons* with dementia will enjoy creating and looking at this collage and celebrating the color blue.

The Basics

- Blue 22" × 28" poster board (any size will do), cut in half (cut lengthwise for an interesting long collage)
- White school glue
- Glue gun (for items that are heavier than paper)
- Scissors
- Magazines
- Miscellaneous collage items that are blue (e.g., craft sticks, tissue or construction paper, silk flowers, glitter, yarn)
- Black and white construction paper

Look through magazines and cut out pictures of blue things, including words or letters, a bluebird, a blue lake, a blue dress, blue jeans, a model with blue eyes, a blue gemstone, blue wallpaper and fabric, and so forth.

Lay out pictures on poster board. Mat some of them with black or white construction paper to intensify the blue colors. Glue down with white glue.

Lay out collage items. Glue down with glue gun. Set aside to let dry. You can do this project in 1 day or spread it out over time.

Variation: This activity works with any color!

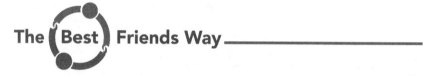

The (Best) Friends Way

Life Story: Know each *person's* favorite color for discussion, especially if it is blue. Gather collage items that speak to a *person's* life story, such as blue ribbons or certificates. Who has blue eyes in the group? Who likes to wear blue jeans?

Music: Have the lyrics to "Alice Blue Gown," "Blue Moon," or "Lavender Blue," and burst into song while looking at your blue collage.

Humor: Look for humorous pictures to cut out.

Old Sayings: "Once in a blue moon" (a blue moon is the second full moon in any month). "Blue Monday." "Something old, something new, something borrowed, something blue." "Feeling blue." "Ol' Blue Eyes" (Frank Sinatra).

Old Skills: Organizing the items that have been collected is an old skill.

Sensory: Explore the various shades of blue on the finished piece.

Spirituality: Assign spiritual names to the collages, such as "comfort," "sky," "clear water," and so forth. Obtain pictures of the famed Blue Mosque in Istanbul.

Late Dementia: The ability to identify colors often remains intact long into the disease.

Conversation: Reminisce: "Gil, have you ever had a 'Blue Monday' candy bar?" Ponder: "Miriam, is the "Blue" Danube River really blue?" Be playful: "Mike, you have beautiful blue eyes." Ask for help: "Marian, is my suit jacket dark blue or black? I have trouble telling."

The Basics

- Balloon, blown up to the size of an orange to fit in the palm of the hand
- Small paper plate for paint
- Three colors of paint in squirt bottles (small ketchup-style bottles work well)
- White paper
- Newspapers

Lay out newspapers to cover work area. Squirt three colors of paint (the size of a dime each) onto the paper plate so that the sides are touching and the paint will run together.

Take the balloon and use it to stamp into the paint, and then press the balloon directly onto the paper repeatedly until the page is covered with differing intensities of color. Repeat steps if necessary. The tied end of the balloon is useful, too, because it creates a different effect. Mat the paintings on contrasting paper, and hang on the walls for decoration.

Variations: This is a good technique for festive greeting cards. (See Volume One, Creating One-of-a-Kind Greeting Cards, p. 77.) Sprinkle on a little glitter to add sparkle.

Balloon Prints

We all enjoy splashes of color, and balloon prints are one way to make a colorful design. *Persons* with dementia may delight in the elegance of the intricately mixed colors that are created by this simple process.

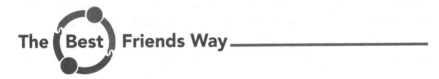

The (Best) Friends Way

Life Story: What are the *person's* memories of balloons? Check whether anyone has ever flown in a hot-air balloon. Did the *person* ever paint for a hobby or engage in other creative pursuits?

The Arts: Look at the designs and figures in this print and give them names.

Music: "Up, Up and Away," by The Fifth Dimension.

Humor: Laugh about trying to catch a water balloon without breaking it.

Sensory: The feel of the balloon and bright colors are stimulating. Listen to the squeaky sound of the balloon.

Late Dementia: Sometimes it helps to lay hand over hand for a *person* who may be confused by this unusual use of a balloon. This is an art activity that is especially good for those with a hand tremor; a steady hand is not necessary.

Conversation: Ask for a long-term memory: "Gladys, do you remember the first time you saw a balloon?" Create names for the paintings: "Alise, what shall we call this beautiful painting?" Ask a safe question: "Helene, do balloons remind you of birthdays?" Encourage simple choices: "Which color should we use, orange?"

Bean Mosaics

Dried beans can be used to make a simple mosaic that repeats the hip style of the 1970s. *Persons* with dementia often enjoy the repetitive process of making a pattern with an unusual art material, such as dried beans.

The Basics

- Variety of dried beans
- White glue
- Pencil
- Cardboard
- Colored sand
- Craft sealer

Sort beans by type. Draw a design on the cardboard; a landscape or a starburst works well. With white glue, cover a section of the design on the cardboard where the beans are to go. Arrange the beans on the glued surface. Use various types of beans to add texture to the design. Alternate a section of large beans against a section of smaller beans. Use dark and light colors for added variation. Sprinkle colored sand between the beans. Let dry completely. Spray with craft sealer.

Tip: See Planning Group, p. 163, for sorting the beans, and Sorting with Meaning, p. 191.

The 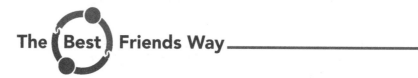 Best Friends Way

Life Story: Know about the region where the *person* is from and the types of beans grown and eaten there. Did anyone have a beanbag chair years ago? Is anyone a vegetarian who eats beans as his or her major source of protein? Did someone grow beans in his or her backyard garden or family farm?

Humor: Bring in some jumping beans for a good laugh!

Old Sayings: Read the story *Jack and the Beanstalk.* "That's not worth a hill of beans."

Old Skills: Sorting beans and looking for stones to remove is an old skill for anyone who has done kitchen work.

Sensory: Create a pattern in the design for visual interest. Feel the different sizes and shapes of the beans.

Spirituality: Enjoy a conversation about how seeds represent new beginnings and growth.

Early Dementia: The *person* may be encouraged to make a more complicated design.

Late Dementia: Rub hands along the surface of the completed mosaic to enjoy the texture, after the glue has dried.

Conversation: Reminisce: "Greta, you grew up on a farm; did your family ever grow and dry beans?" Reminisce: "Toby, my favorite beans to eat when I was growing up were pinto beans. Did your family eat pinto beans?" Talk about common travels: "Justin, did you get to taste the wonderful refried beans when you were in Mexico?" Discuss a superstition: "Cabby, is it true that people in New Orleans eat black-eyed peas on New Year's Eve for good luck?"

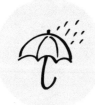

An ounce of prevention . . .

Supervise closely to make sure that no one eats the raw beans.

The Basics _____

- Clay, air-drying type
- Rolling pin
- Small newspaper stack, at least ½" thick
- Table knife or wire for cutting clay
- Ruler
- Permanent marker

Warm up clay in your hands, then roll it out until it is smooth and approximately ½" thick. Measure 1" squares with the ruler; mark straight lines by creating an indentation in the clay.

Cut out the squares with the knife. Keep the cuts straight by cutting against the ruler. Lay out squares on slightly dampened newspaper or any flat surface to air-dry for at least 24 hours, or according to package directions. When completely dry, use a marker to make one letter of the alphabet on each tile (see Volume One, Working with Letters, p. 99, for ideas on how to use the letters).

Tip: Make extra vowels and commonly used consonants (you can use the breakdown of letters in a Scrabble game as a model).

Variation: Make free-form sculptures.

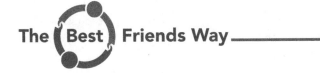

The (Best) Friends Way _____

Life Story: Identify words and lists that may be of interest to the *person*, such as family names, places that he or she has lived, favorite words, or simple poems that may be spelled out. Has someone ever worked on a crafts or home improvement project relating to tiles?

Exercise: Working with clay is good exercise for the hands, especially for those with arthritis.

Humor: Make a tile with a smiley face to place in unexpected words for fun.

Old Skills: Warming up the clay with your hands is similar to kneading bread.

Sensory: It feels good to mold clay in the hands once it has become soft.

Spirituality: Spell out words that evoke a feeling of spirituality: inspiration, peace, tranquility, serene, faith, dream, love, beauty, nature, transcendent, and so forth.

Early Dementia: If the *person* would like to make other shapes with the clay, then encourage creativity. Play an impromptu game of Scrabble.

Late Dementia: Celebrate a *person's* remaining skills. Encourage rolling the clay with the rolling pin.

Conversation: Ask an opinion: "Ellery, how do you think we should make this clay smooth?" Draw attention to the spelling of simple words: "Some people spell their name M-A-E, and some spell it M-A-Y. Which way do you spell yours?" Ponder: "I wonder where this clay came from."

Making Clay Tile Letters

Spelling words with a set of letters that are handmade and tactually appealing is a fun way to spend time with a friend. *Persons* with dementia enjoy making this simple project because the tiles can be used over and over again.

An ounce of prevention . . .

Have all supplies ready before you begin. Sit down with the person and give all of your attention to creating together, not getting up for distractions such as the telephone.

Crayon Melts

The many bright colors of crayons make them an attractive art medium, yet it is challenging to find simple projects using crayons that do not feel childish. *Persons* with dementia will enjoy creating these unusual art pieces with melted crayons.

The Basics

- Plain white paper
- Electric pancake griddle
- Old crayons, papers removed
- Hand pencil/crayon sharpener

Sharpen crayons to make shavings. Place shavings of many different colors on the white paper.

Place the paper with the shavings on the pancake griddle set to the lowest setting. Watch the crayon shavings melt. Remove paper when the crayon shavings are melted. Lay flat to cool. Sign and name the colorful designs for display.

This activity validates the value of being frugal and using old crayons to make something special.

Variation: A cheese grater may be used to shave the crayons.

The (Best) Friends Way

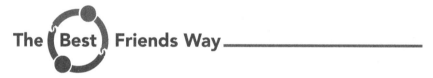

Life Story: Does someone recall using crayons as a child? Did the *person* use the crayons down to the smallest stub? How many of us can recall our sadness when a crayon broke too soon? Who remembers when there were only eight crayons to a box versus the big collections today?

Exercise: Shaving the crayon is a fine motor exercise.

Old Skills: Sharpening a crayon is like sharpening a pencil in school.

Sensory: The texture of the crayons is smooth in the beginning, then it breaks up when the crayon gets shredded. When it melts, it becomes smooth again.

Early Dementia: Try to plan the designs a bit by using a pencil to draw a loose outline of a butterfly on the paper, then arrange the crayon shavings on the paper according to the outline.

Late Dementia: The *person* can enjoy the social group and the bright colors.

Conversation: Explain the unusual process: "Alma, let's take the papers off these broken crayons so that we can use them for the melted crayon paintings." Ponder: "Irene, I wonder who first made crayons. I think they've been around a long time." Be surprised: "This crayon is called 'Mulberry.' Isn't that a funny name for a color?"

An ounce of prevention . . .

Supervise closely to ensure that no one gets burned on the griddle. Persons with short-term memory loss may forget that it is hot! The freshly melted crayon wax is also hot to the touch, so be careful moving the paper before it cools.

The Basics ─────────────

- Styrofoam eggs (available from craft stores)
- Tissue paper or wrapping paper (decorative, with varying colors)
- White glue (or other decoupage sealer)
- Paint brush
- Small plate for glue

Introduce the activity by describing the origins of the word *decoupage.* Tear tissue paper into small pieces, approximately 1" × 1". If using wrapping paper, then cut out small designs. Paint glue onto a small area of the egg using a brush. Place paper pieces on the egg on top of the glue, smoothing out wrinkles with the fingertips; continue all the way around the egg to cover the entire surface. Tissue paper should be overlapped some. Brush on sealer and let dry. Fill a pretty bowl with the decoupage eggs for a centerpiece.

Tip: Save egg cartons to hold the completed decoupage eggs for drying.

Variation: Design an egg tree using a leafless branch of a tree mounted on a piece of driftwood or weathered board. Attach ribbon to the egg using a straight pin. Hang the eggs in the tree.

Decoupage Eggs

Decoupage, from the French word *decouper,* meaning to cut out, is an ancient art. This activity is great for making year-round decorations and gifts. A *person* with dementia will enjoy the socialization of this adult-oriented alternative to dying Easter eggs.

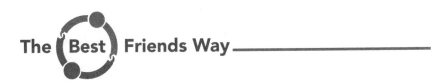

The (Best) Friends Way ─────────────

Life Story: Find out whether the *person* has ever raised chickens for eggs, enjoyed decorating eggs for Easter, or made decoupage pictures. Has anyone ever had pickled dove's eggs? Did anyone study French in school?

Exercise: Painting and gluing are good exercises for the wrist and hand.

Humor: Laugh about trying to hard-boil an ostrich egg.

Old Saying: "Don't count your chickens before they're hatched." "Which came first . . . the chicken or the egg?"

Sensory: Feel the smooth texture of the eggs, before and after decoupage.

Spirituality: The egg is a symbol of new life. There are so many special miracles in nature.

Late Dementia: After the decoupage eggs are dry, they provide a good size and shape to hold in the hand and admire.

Conversation: Encourage participation: "Delora, did your birthday gift come wrapped in that paper? Would you like to make a keepsake out of it?" Try a question from long-term memory: "Mike, did you ever enjoy an Easter egg hunt?" Explore history: "Albert, do you think Marie Antoinette practiced the art of decoupage?" Offer information: "Cindy, I know that your grandparents were from China. Did you know that ancient Chinese artists used decoupage techniques to decorate lanterns?"

Embossing

Embossing is a traditional approach to creating art that is simple and elegant and involves raised ink. *Persons* with dementia enjoy a quick result to their efforts and the flexibility to make art as simple or as detailed as they choose.

The Basics

- Embossing powder (available at craft stores)
- Heat tool (available at craft stores)
- Colored ink pad
- Rubber stamps of letters, flowers, animals, or geometric shapes
- Cardstock
- Small bowl to catch excess embossing powder

Lay out cardstock flat on a table. Press the rubber stamp onto the ink pad, and then press down firmly and evenly onto the cardstock. Lift stamp straight up.

Sprinkle embossing powder onto the wet ink, then tap from side to side to ensure that all of the wet ink is covered with powder. Tilt paper to the side to let excess powder run off into the small bowl. Turn on the heat tool and apply heat to the powdered ink (manufacturers will often have more detailed instructions on the heat tool).

Clean the stamps when finished so they will last a long time. This process may be used to create bookmarks, greeting cards, or personalized stationery.

Variation: Using black ink on light paper enables you to color in the stamped design with felt tip markers, colored pencils, watercolors, or chalk.

The 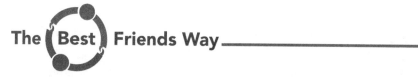 Best Friends Way

Life Story: Find stamps that fit the interests of the *person*. There are stamps on every subject: fishing, floral, whimsical, holiday, traditional, spiritual, and so forth. Did anyone ever have fancy embossed letterhead or notecards for correspondence?

Sensory: The raised lines of the design offer a quick, gentle tactile experience.

Early Dementia: Stamps may be layered for a more interesting design. Various methods of art can be used together for a mixed media look, such as stamping, embossing, painting, pen and ink or markers, tissue paper, and collage. All of these may be done on fabric instead of paper or done on recycled paintings. Use your imagination.

Late Dementia: Just stamp designs on paper and skip the embossing process to make the project simple. Stamping is good for *persons* in late dementia because there is a quick reward of a design on a page.

Conversation: Observe together: "My goodness, George, look what talented artists we are!" Suggest an idea: "Let's use the rubber stamp to stamp out a bunch of strawberries, then we'll draw a nice bowl to hold them all. Did you ever think we could draw such a wonderful bowl of strawberries?" Reminisce: "Loretta, did you ever have a box of embossed stationery?" Ask for help: "Marvin, will you help me choose a design for this card that I am making for Donna's birthday?" Ponder: "Beulah, I wonder how this powder makes the ink rise up like that."

An ounce of prevention . . .

Supervise the use of the embossing tool because it can get hot.

The Basics _____

- Different colors or patterns of fabric
- White glue
- Iron
- Scissors

If the fabric is wrinkled, then use a warm iron to press flat. Cut a piece of fabric that is 8" × 10" for the background. Cut out the flower pieces. Make three different-sized shapes for layering. The shapes may be similar or totally different.

Assemble the layers. Lay out the background piece first. Layer the flower pieces, largest on bottom. Glue wrong side of fabric, and place on background. Continue until each piece is adhered. For a finishing option, laminate it for a mat. Be sure to discuss fabric selections and give participants choices so that they may know that the project is their creation.

Variation: Interfacing from a fabric store may be used to hold the fabric layers together rather than glue for a smoother look.

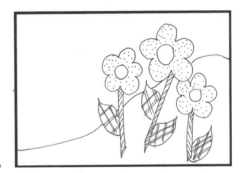

Fabric Flowers

The best projects are ones that can be shown off and enjoyed or given as gifts. *Persons* with dementia will enjoy this easy, tactile, and colorful project that uses fabric to create a picture of flowers.

The (Best) Friends Way _____

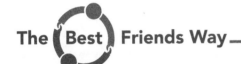

Life Story: Find out if *persons* enjoyed going to fabric stores, sewed, or collected patterns. Did a mother or grandmother make their clothes?

The Arts: Sew the fabric pieces together to make a wall hanging (see Wall Tapestry, p. 137).

Humor: Joke about wacky fabric.

Old Sayings: "A stitch in time saves nine."

Old Skills: Working with fabric is an old skill for many: sorting, cutting, planning, arranging.

Sensory: Touch the different textures of fabric. Use brightly colored fabrics for eye appeal.

Early Dementia: A *person* in early dementia could assist in the ironing of the fabric pieces.

Late Dementia: A *person* in late stage may enjoy sorting the fabric or folding it.

Conversation: Talk about handmade clothing and quilts. Talk about different types of fabric and which type *persons* like to wear. Reminisce: "My mother had a dress made of fabric like this." Ask an opinion: "Mrs. Temple, do these two prints go well together?" Joke: "If you had a dress made out of this, they would see you coming a mile away!"

Painting Tile Trivets

Many of us have painted on paper. Painting on tiles is a novel experience. *Persons* with dementia will enjoy this fresh approach and will be able to see their artistic achievement in a dramatic way.

The Basics

- White ceramic tiles, matte finished (4" × 4" is a good size)
- Tempera or acrylic paint
- Any kind of brushes, stamps, or sponges
- Craft sealer spray (available at craft stores)
- Felt pads (small circles), with adhesive on one side (available at craft stores)

Make sure that the tile is clean and dry before use. Let everyone examine the tile to explore the texture. Choose colors for the design.

Using the brush, stamps, or sponges, apply paint to the tile. Explain that the paint may be applied to the tile any way they want, using any color paint.

Let dry. Spray sealer on painting. Let dry again. Apply felt pads to the bottom four corners.

The finished product makes a wonderful gift for a family member, friend, or staff. It can be used in the kitchen as a hot plate or coaster (smaller tile sizes) or in the garden for decoration.

Tip: Some *persons* may enjoy signing their creation on the bottom with a felt-tipped marker.

The 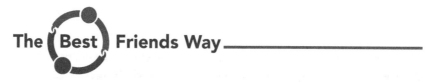 Best Friends Way

Life Story: Did anyone collect unusual tiles? Has anyone seen the intricate mosaic tile designs on European churches and castles, such as the Blue Mosque in Istanbul or the Sistine Chapel in Rome?

Sensory: The smooth, slick texture of the unpainted tile is interesting.

Spirituality: Religious symbols, such as a bell, a star, or a cross, can be incorporated into the activity.

Early Dementia: The *person* might want to make a more specific design, such as a family coat of arms, favorite pet, or self-portrait.

Late Dementia: A beautiful painting on the tile may be created by minimal effort with a sponge or a balloon.

Conversation: Ask an opinion: "Shirley, should we use red and yellow to match your kitchen?" Compliment: "Nora, I love your black figures. They look like a flock of birds to me." Examine the tile: "Mollie, feel how heavy this tile is. Any guesses about how much it weighs?" Discuss: "Jim, do you think a coaster like this would help us protect the wood table?"

The Basics _____

- Two 11" × 14" sheets of paper
- Tempera paint in squirt bottles
- Newspaper

Lay out newspapers and place one sheet of the plain paper on the newspaper. Partners take turns applying paint to the same piece of paper. Be careful not to put paint too close to the edge.

Lay the second piece of paper directly on top of the one that has the paint on it. Both partners lay all four hands on the paper and gently rub it so that the paint gets spread around. Lift off the top sheet of paper and find two of the same paintings!

During the process, take time to talk about colors, texture, and the project. Enjoy the nonverbal touch.

Note that the pieces are often beautiful but abstract. Discuss the meaning of the pieces and name them. Encourage the artists to sign their work.

Variation: The partner technique may be used with markers or pencils or pens, except there will be only one painting.

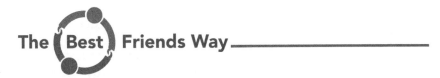

The (Best) Friends Way _____

Life Story: Think about the partners in the group. Who has a partner in marriage, a twin, brothers and sisters, best friends, business partners? Has anyone been a painter or artist? Is anyone good with picking colors, or does anyone have a good eye for design?

Humor: "We are partners in crime!"

Old Sayings: "They say, 'Two heads are better than one.' How about two hands?" "Many hands make light work."

Sensory: Hand over hand is a good way to include touch in the activity.

Spirituality: Being together and creating together give us support and the feeling that we are not alone.

Early Dementia: This is an open-ended painting that may be done in as much detail as a *person* desires.

Late Dementia: Such a simple technique produces fantastic results.

Conversation: Relate the activity to other life experiences: "Agnes, what other jobs can you think of that require two partners to complete?" Speculate: "What do you think this looks like?" Laugh about a saying: "Lydia, I heard that it takes two to tango." Ponder: "Melody, I wonder what 'partners' really means. Let's look it up in the dictionary." Celebrate: "Hope, we have paintings just alike. We must be twins."

We all enjoy having a friend with whom we can share activities. *Persons* with dementia thrive on having a partner to share this rewarding, surprisingly simple art project that results in a "limited edition" of two identical prints.

Rubbings

Rubbing involves laying a sheet of paper on an object and then rubbing the paper with a crayon or pencil until the likeness is reproduced. Many individuals have enjoyed rubbings from something as simple as coins to more elaborate brass rubbings of famous markers or plaques around the world. *Persons* with dementia relate to this activity in part because of its historic roots and adult feel.

The Basics

- Plain white paper or black paper that goes well with gold or silver crayons
- Textured items: coins, burlap, leaves, brass nameplates, brass plates from trophies, raised lettering on old books, wood boards, or sandpaper
- Crayons or pencils

Lay the textured item flat on the table. Place the white or black paper on top. Color over the textured item with the crayon. Use even strokes to fill in the entire area to pick up the texture.

Tip: Choose items with well-defined textures so that the rubbing will pick it up easily. Some coins may be too small, but large coins, such as half dollars, work well.

Variation: Use different colors.

The 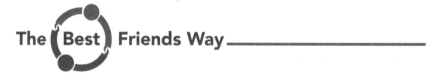 Best Friends Way

Life Story: Choose textured items that relate to a *person's* interests. For example, a coin collector might like to use interesting coins, a nature lover might like to use different-shaped leaves, a seamstress might like to use lace, and so forth. Use an award or a plaque that belongs to the *person* to show off a past achievement in his or her rubbing. Find out if someone ever did a brass rubbing of an ancient monument and ask the family to bring in the piece if still available.

Old Sayings: "You rub me the wrong way!"

Sensory: Begin by exploring the materials. Run your hand along the textured item to feel the bumps or ridges that will create the design. This texture contrasts with the smoothness of the paper. The round, smooth crayon adds yet another sensory experience.

Spirituality: Many individuals do religiously themed brass rubbings or rubbings from cathedrals and churches.

Late Dementia: This simple motion of the crayon filling in an area on the page can feel satisfying because you can see the results from a small effort.

Conversation: Recognize a *person's* accomplishments: "Eugene, I see that you have won an award for designing machinery! Let's make a special work of art from the nameplate on your plaque!" Encourage participation: "Robert, would you color on this side to see what will show through?" Reminisce: "Joan, I heard that you made some beautiful brass rubbings when you visited Oxford, England."

The Basics ————————————————

- White eggshells
- 8" × 10" cardboard
- Craft knife
- White glue
- Paper towels
- Dark-color paint
- Paper bag
- Rolling pin
- Bleach
- Vinegar
- Clear varnish sealer
- 4" × 6" photo
- Paintbrushes

We never have enough picture frames. *Persons* with dementia will enjoy making something unique and useful, such as picture frames made from eggshells!

Prepare the base of the mat by cutting a 4" × 6" section out of the center of an 8" × 10" cardboard with a craft knife. This can be done ahead of time by the planning group (see Planning Group, p. 163).

To prepare eggshells, soak them in bleach for an hour. This removes the membranes. Rinse with vinegar. Lay out on doubled paper towels to dry. When dry, put shells in a paper bag, then roll with a rolling pin until the shells are crushed into small pieces.

Lay out newspapers over workspace. Paint one side of the cardboard with a dark-color paint. Allow to dry. Water down the glue just enough to make it easy to spread, then apply to painted side of the mat. Sprinkle the eggshells onto the wet glued surface. Repeat as necessary to evenly cover the mat. Allow to dry. Seal with a clear varnish sealer. Allow to dry. Choose a picture for your frame and tape it to the mat.

Tip: Combine this activity with the pictures that were taken in the photography activity (see Photo Shoot, p. 50).

Variation: A premade picture mat could be used instead of cutting your own.

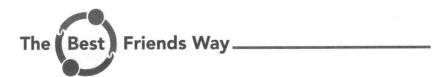

The (Best) Friends Way ————————————————

Life Story: Did anyone raise chickens and gather the eggs each morning before school? Who in the group likes egg salad sandwiches or deviled eggs? Who in the group took lots of pictures while on vacation, and who did not?

Old Sayings: "Don't put all your eggs in one basket."

Old Skills: Anyone who has used a rolling pin for baking may have ideas about how to roll the pin.

Sensory: Feel the rough texture by touching the dry finished product. Observe the contrast between the dark background and the white eggshells.

Spirituality: Talk about family and friends in a framed photo.

Late Dementia: A *person* in late dementia can sometimes roll the rolling pin over the bag to crush the eggshells.

Conversation: Ask some easy questions: "What makes brown eggs?" "How do you like your eggs to be cooked?" "Have you ever seen a baby bird peck its way out of the shell?" Remember a *person's* hobby: "Aubrey, I know that you love photography. Won't your black-and-white photos look nice in this frame?"

Newspaper Art

Newspaper advertisements, photos, cartoons, and headlines can inspire art projects, whether creating collages or making origami folded cranes. *Persons* with dementia can help find interesting ideas from something as simple as a discarded newspaper.

The Basics

- Newspaper, preferably a Sunday edition with comics or a *USA Today* for its rich, colorful visuals
- Crayons
- Markers
- Scissors
- Liquid starch
- Glue

Search the newspaper for an interesting photograph, then find words or letters from the newspaper to add a new caption. Paste the picture and the new caption on a piece of construction paper and add a title, or frame a picture with poster board and paste descriptive words and phrases on the frame.

Make a collage from pictures, headlines, comics, or advertisements. Choose a theme, such as my favorite things, sports events, cars for sale, nature, or stock market news. Use the newspaper to make papier mâché and decoupage material. Use the Sunday funnies to wrap presents; add a bright bow for a finishing touch.

Variation: Make a large origami object by using the colored comics. For instructions to make a paper crane, go to www.sadako.com/fold/folding.html.

The 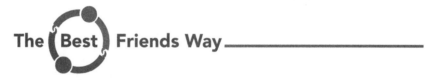 Best Friends Way

Life Story: The collage can be designed with each *person's* life story in mind. Choose all of the things that a *person* likes, or choose pictures that relate to favorite memories. Who loves looking through the paper?

Humor: Read the comics and experiment with rewriting one for more laughs.

Old Skills: Ask a *person* to read to the group the caption of a picture or a brief account of an interesting article.

Sensory: Clip a recipe to be made and tasted later.

Early Dementia: *Persons* can work on their own to find words and phrases that describe the picture. They may also be interested in the art of origami.

Late Dementia: *Persons* are often content to thumb through or hold the newspaper.

Conversation: Recall a *person's* interest: "Colleen, you are the best pie maker. Let's choose some of these pictures of fruits for making fruit pies." Compliment: "Ed, I'll bet your horse could jump even higher than the one here in this picture." Ponder: "Virginia, it says here, 'A picture is worth a thousand words.' I wonder what that means?" Ask for help: "Colleen, I need for you to crease this sheet of paper along this fold. Thanks. That is a big help."

An ounce of prevention . . .

Remove sections of the paper that contain unusually violent or otherwise disturbing information.

The Basics _____

- Popsicle sticks or coffee stirrers (enough for each *person* to have nine sticks)
- Construction paper of various colors
- Glue or glue gun
- Magic markers

Research a few facts about some famous architects, such as Frank Lloyd Wright or Thomas Jefferson, who designed the famous house Monticello. Obtain books with pictures of architects and their creations. One thing that great builders have in common is their creative thinking, enabling them to see new ways to approach a project. Ask certain *persons* to read some of the researched facts about designs and builders, and encourage any comments.

Let *persons* choose the color of paper that they like the best. Provide each *person* with nine sticks. Encourage creativity by asking each *person* to arrange the sticks in a design on his or her paper. The sticks are to remain unbroken but can lie flat or be three-dimensional. When the design is chosen, glue the sticks in place. Talk about each creation and the many ways in which *persons* chose to arrange their sticks to make the design.

Variation: Use small sticks and twigs glued to construction paper or cloth for an interesting design. This is especially effective when used with an outdoor topic, such as camping or hiking.

Stick Design

We are designers by nature. *Persons* with dementia may be interested in noting how many different designs can be made with nine sticks. This is a good example of a simple activity that is designed to be more adult.

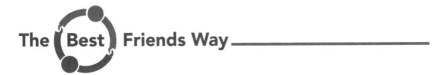

The (Best) Friends Way _____

Life Story: Does anyone have a background in construction or design? Did anyone spend time in school doodling with line drawings? Did anyone build a house? As a child, did anyone play pick up sticks (or pick-a-stick).

The Arts: Give each *person* an opportunity to comment on his or her design. Encourage *persons* to title and sign their design to be hung in an art interest corner.

Humor: Playfully tease the *person* about being a famous designer.

Old Skills: This activity may remind *persons* of playing Pick Up Sticks.

Sensory: Handling, arranging, and gluing the sticks are tactile experiences.

Early Dementia: *Persons* can help research the facts about architectural design and read some of this information to the group.

Late Dementia: *Persons* may want to hold or count the sticks.

Conversation: With surprise: "Minot, you dropped your sticks on your paper, and look at your design. It is amazing!" Compliment: "Mimi, that looks like the Leaning Tower of Pisa." Seek information: "Jacob, did you study design before you opened your flower shop?" Compliment: "You created a tepee. That is very creative."

Watercolor Techniques

Many *persons* with dementia can find joy, improved focus, self-esteem, enhanced language, and creativity through the medium of art. These simple, nontraditional watercolor techniques yield surprising patterns, often stimulating unexpected memories, emotions, and artistic interpretations as a *person* creates his or her own watercolor painting.

The Basics

- Watercolor paper, approximately 4" × 6" or 5" × 8" in size
- Watercolor paints
- Plastic wrap
- Eye dropper
- Paintbrushes
- Water
- Rubbing alcohol
- Kosher salt

Create a quiet work environment that is free of clutter to avoid distraction. Wet the front and the back of a postcard-size watercolor paper (by wetting the back, the paper will not curl). Use a wide paintbrush and water. Paper should not be too wet nor too dry. Apply watercolor paints (either one color or a variety of colors) to entire paper.

  Optional finishing techniques:
- Crumple plastic wrap, press it firmly to paper, and allow to dry.
- Using an eye dropper, drip drops of alcohol onto paints.
- Sprinkle kosher salt onto the wet paper.
- Tilt the paper toward the top or bottom and allow the paints to run.

Submitted by Karen Zwicke, MA, CCC-SLP, Santa Barbara, CA.

The 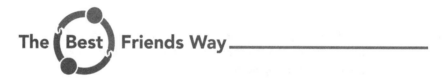 Best Friends Way

Life Story: What connection does the *person* have to art? Has the *person* enjoyed art as an observer? Did he or she have to create displays or designs as part of his or her job? Would the *person* describe him- or herself as "creative"?

The Arts: Explore artists who have used watercolors or unique techniques with paint.

Exercise: Painting, crumpling the plastic wrap, squeezing the eye dropper, and sprinkling the salt exercise the fine motor skills.

Old Skills: Using an eye dropper, sprinkling salt, and tearing off sheets of plastic wrap all are old skills.

Sensory: Notice how the salt interacts with the watercolors, distributing the paint as the salt dissolves. Hear the sound of and the feel of the crumpling plastic wrap.

Early Dementia: Encourage the *person* to create a series of watercolor prints using the four techniques. Discuss each one with the *person*.

Late Dementia: Encourage the *person* to hold the paper up and watch the paint run.

Conversation: Marvel together: "Robin, I love your choice of colors." Encourage participation: "Jacob, will you help me crumple this plastic wrap for the painting?" Suppress the urge to label the painting. Instead, allow the *person* time to interpret the results. If necessary, offer gentle prompts, such as, "What is this?" or "What is happening here?" When finished, ask the *person* to title the painting.

The Basics _____

- Plain white paper
- Tempera paint, in an open container or tray
- String, 10-ply cotton, cut in 18" lengths
- Newspaper

Cover the work area with newspaper. Take one sheet of paper and lay it flat on the table. Holding one end of the string in your hand, dip the length of the string, except the end in your hand, into the paint. Lift the paint-coated string straight up, and dangle it down onto the paper. Place the clean end of the string toward the bottom of the paper.

Fold the paper in half, with the painted string inside. Lay one hand gently over the paper to hold it down while you gently pull the string from the unpainted end all the way out of the paper. Discard the string. Open the paper and view your design.

Variations: Use a second string dipped in paint of a different color. Try white paint on dark paper. Lay the string on the paper and let it dry there for an interesting effect.

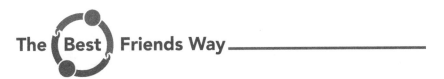

The (Best) Friends Way _____

Life Story: Who likes to try new things? Has the *person* enjoyed good eye–hand coordination in the past? Did he or she ever play a string instrument?

Humor: Have you ever played with a cat using a string? They'll play for hours!

Old Sayings: "She is high strung." "Don't string me along."

Sensory: Pass around the ball of string. The feel of the string beneath your hand provides a unique sensory experience.

Early Dementia: Encourage the *person* to plan and/or help lead the activity.

Late Dementia: Hand the end of the string to the *person* and ask him or her to help as needed.

Conversation: Encourage participation: "David, move your string around in the paint until it is all red. That's right. Now we are ready to move to the next step." Share something in common: "Look, Jenny, we both chose the orange paint." Laugh: "Lucy, I thought when I pulled the string something would pop up!" Make an observation: "Lois, this looks like an iris to me. What do you think?"

Painting with String

This painting project is much less intimidating than using a paint-brush on a blank page. *Persons* with dementia can make unusual paintings without a paintbrush by using this simple, structured technique with string.

Sponge Painting

All of us have worked with sponges during our life for cleaning up the counter, doing the dishes, or washing the car. This activity involves *persons* with dementia in a simple art project using this everyday object.

The Basics

- Different colors of paint
- White or colored painting paper
- Small paper plate or other tray to hold paint
- Sponges (can be plain, cut into shapes, or precut)

Feel the texture of the sponges to explore the shapes. Place a small amount of paint on the paper plate. Lay the sponge flat to cover with the paint. Press the painted side of the sponge onto the paper a few times to create lighter and darker images of the sponge shape.

Tip: Use paper that is thick enough to hold the paint; the weight of construction paper works well for a thin coat of paint. The planning group can precut sponge shapes (see Planning Group, p. 163).

Variations:
- Use a balloon that is blown up to the size of a small apple. Use the balloon in place of the sponge in the above directions (see Balloon Prints, p. 121).
- Use a potato stamp. Cut a potato in half, then carve a shape out of the flat surface, such as a flower, a heart, or a square. Follow the process for sponge painting above.

The 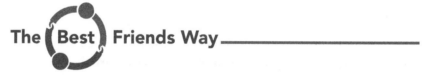 Best Friends Way

Life Story: Did anyone in the group enjoy diving or swimming in the ocean, where they might have seen sea sponges? Is anyone in the group a "neatnik," someone who always kept his or her place immaculate (using a cleaner with a sponge)? Has someone used a sponge for hanging wallpaper?

Old Skills: Some *persons* will relate to their past use of sponges for household work.

Sensory: Feel the texture of the sponge before paint is applied to it.

Early Dementia: *Persons* with early dementia often have bursts of creativity. This is a satisfying project for them.

Late Dementia: A *person* in late dementia can handle the sponges with hand on hand prompting.

Conversation: Ask for help: "Mary, do you think it's better to clean with a sponge or a good rag?" Ask for information: "Tony, did you know that there are natural sea sponges as well as manufactured ones? Which do you think are better?" Encourage participation: "Billy, you have such a good eye. Will you help me get this project started?"

The Basics

- Large piece of solid-color fabric
- Fabric with various designs and textures
- Scissors
- Needle and thread
- Pencil or pen

Begin by sketching the design of the tapestry onto the solid piece of fabric. The design can be abstract or a specific scene. Decide which of the other fabrics you will use for each part. Cut the fabric to create the design. Sew the pieces into place.

Tip: Some design shops or home stores may donate fabric sample books for use in the project.

Variation: Use glue or iron-on fabric instead of sewing.

The (Best) Friends Way

Life Story: Create a design that relates to the *person's* life story, hobbies, or interests. Examples include cats, life on the farm, New York landscapes, fall colors, or other topics or themes of interest to the *person.*

The Arts: Discuss famous tapestries or try to re-create a famed painting for your tapestry, such as Vincent van Gogh's "Starry Night."

Music: Sing a song together as you work on piecing together the tapestry.

Exercise: Cutting and sewing are great exercise for the hands.

Old Sayings: "A stitch in time saves nine."

Old Skills: Sewing may be an old skill for many. The rhythm of sewing by hand can be relaxing.

Sensory: Choose fabrics that not only are colorful and bright with patterns but also have varied texture so as to stimulate the senses.

Spirituality: Create a wall tapestry out of biblical/spiritual themes. Look at a book of old tapestries related to religion, or discuss religious garments and vestments.

Early Dementia: Take a day trip to visit community museums or churches to admire their wall tapestries.

Late Dementia: Enjoy handling the fabric and the companionship.

Conversation: Compliment: "Jo, I like the fabric that you chose for the dove." Ask for help: "Would you mind holding the fabric while I cut it?" Reminisce: "I used to have a shirt made out of fabric just like this. Did you ever wear anything with these colors?" Encourage participation: "Matt, you are so good at sewing. Would you sew these pieces together?"

Wall Tapestry

Tapestry is an ancient art, and many of us have seen historic tapestries in museums, cathedrals, or castles. A wall tapestry usually covers a theme and can almost be read like a book. It can also provide visual cues for conversations and reminiscing. This activity encourages the creation of a wall tapestry to decorate a *person's* home or residential community.

An ounce of prevention . . .

Keep the design simple and provide plenty of supervision with scissors and needles.

A Tree for All Seasons

A bulletin board depicting a tree trunk and branches that change leaves with each season can add a bright spot of warmth to a facility or a home. *Persons* with dementia appreciate this little touch of outdoors being brought to them indoors.

The Basics

- Bulletin board paper in sky blue (purchased from an arts-and-crafts or teachers' supply store)
- Brown craft paper or large sheet of brown cardboard
- Construction paper and/or tissue paper for leaves and/or blossoms
- Scissors and craft knife
- Pencil
- Yard stick or ruler
- Stapler

Cover the bulletin board with sky blue paper for the background using an opened stapler. Lay out the craft paper on a large table. Measure and roughly mark in pencil the size of the bulletin board on the brown craft paper or cardboard to know how large to make the tree. Draw a silhouette of a tree trunk and branches, then cut it out with the scissors and the craft knife. Attach to the bulletin board using the stapler.

In spring, add tiny pieces of balled-up pink tissue paper stapled onto the branches for buds. (The blossoms will be easily detached with a staple remover without damaging the tree.) Add green leaves cut out from construction paper in summer, colorful leaves in autumn, and snow on the bare branches in winter.

Tip: Keep the design simple, uncomplicated, and uncluttered.

Variations: Add a large, white winter moon peeking out from behind the tree or a large, yellow one for an autumn harvest moon. Mountains may be added in the background, cut from purple or navy bulletin board paper. Have fun putting a wise old owl, a bird, or a lost kite in the tree.

The 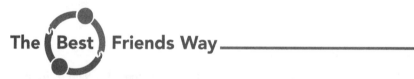 Best Friends Way

Life Story: Anyone who has done paper crafts will enjoy the large project. *Persons* who are interested in nature and the changing of the seasons will be attracted to this project. Did anyone like to climb trees as a child or have fruit trees in his or her backyard?

Arts: Invite a person to read the poem "Trees" by Joyce Kilmer ("I think that I shall never see a poem lovely as a tree . . . ").

Humor: Joke about the pain of raking all those leaves in Fall.

Sensory: The tree against the simple background will be visually stimulating from a good distance because of its size and design.

Early Dementia: Look up the official tree of all fifty states to share with the group.

Late Dementia: A *person* in late stage will enjoy looking at the bulletin board and having simple conversations about the changing seasons.

Conversation: Observe together: "LuAnn, I really like the tree on the bulletin board. I think that it has character just like real trees do. What do you think?" Contemplate: "Mike, is it true that redwood trees live for hundreds of years?" Ask for information: "Jo, is bamboo considered a tree?"

An ounce of prevention . . .

Supervise carefully the cutting of the cardboard tree with the craft knife, or have it done ahead of time.

CHAPTER EIGHT

In the Kitchen

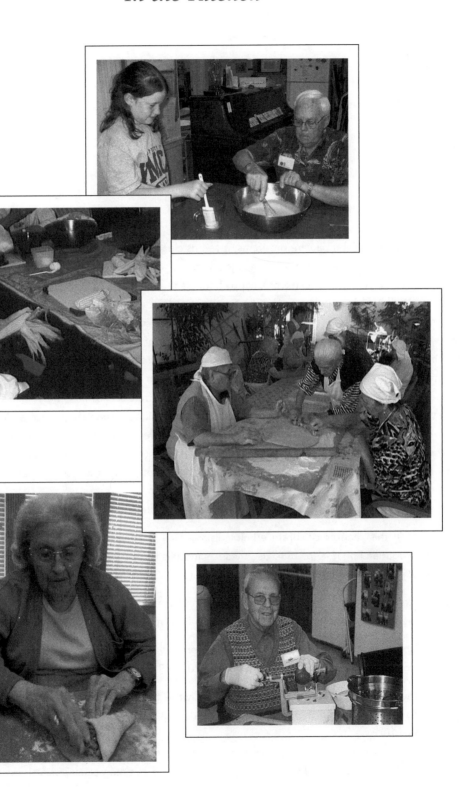

In the Kitchen

For many of us, food is one of the great pleasures of life. Food not only represents survival, but also provides an excuse for socialization, family get-togethers, and celebrating special holidays. For many *persons* with dementia, enjoying a delicious snack or savoring a nice dessert is a highlight of the day.

As we visit various dementia care programs, it seems clear that most are not doing as much as they could do to make the dining experience more enjoyable. On your calendar, do you list a time for "snacks and hydration," or do you offer high tea or a happy hour? Is there a bread-baking machine that is emitting wonderful aromas, or is bread delivered in a plastic bag? Do you take time to set the table in a festive way at least for some meals every week? Is the mealtime filled with conversation or silent? Can residents or day center participants smell the scent and hear the noise of popcorn being made for a movie?

With a little bit of effort, this is one area in which a dementia care program can improve its activity programming. Ask the chef or an interested staff member to do a cooking demonstration. Make some homemade soup, make cookies and cakes, or whip up some fruit smoothies. Try family-style dining, whereby staff members join residents for meals. Watch a nostalgic television show, such as Julia Child, or learn about Greek cooking on one of the food channels. There are many ideas for celebrating good food and good company. When possible, create a more open kitchen space (country kitchens are popular in many new buildings) where residents can get a snack out of the refrigerator or easily observe or take part in some food preparation.

We draw your attention to some of the activities in this chapter:

A few activities in this chapter celebrate ethnic cuisine, such as Making Bunzas (p. 143), Indian Curry (p. 144), and Hungarian Pogacsa (p. 158). Use these as models to design your own programs if you have members of a certain ethnic community in your program (e.g., Greek or Italian cooking).

An Old-Fashioned Tea (p. 152) can be very successful. It evokes old social graces as the ladies wear their hats, a nice table is set, and tea is poured from a vintage teapot.

Crazy for Cookbooks (p. 154) is an activity that many *persons* and staff will enjoy. You can often get an abundance of cookbooks donated if you put out the word.

As with other chapters, we encourage you to tie activities together. Consider I Cast My Vote for . . . (p. 174) to vote on which recipe the group likes best. Make a snack during the day to be eaten in the evening (Chapter 10).

Food-related activities sometimes get derailed out of fears for hygiene. Local health and safety codes vary, but we would argue that with some basic precautions and common sense, most food can be prepared with some involvement from *persons* and still be safe. If that is not possible in your setting, then the program will still benefit from having staff members lead the activities in this chapter.

Tips for staff training: Take time at a staff meeting to encourage staff members to name their favorite foods, reminisce about past holiday meals, discuss a favorite dish from their childhood, or share a recipe from their culture. Note the emotion that accompanies the discussion. Food is often a source of pleasure for staff as much as for *persons* with dementia.

Another way to teach staff about activities and dining is to pick an activity from this chapter and do it together during an in-service. As the activity progresses, draw parallels between the staff experience and what is possible in the dementia care program.

CHAPTER EIGHT ACTIVITIES

The Basics _____

For the filling:
- 1 large head cabbage
- 2 pounds ground beef
- 2 large onions
- Salt and pepper to taste
- Oil, butter, or margarine (½ cup)

For the dough:
- 1 cake yeast
- 2 cups warm milk
- ½ cup sugar
- ½ cup shortening
- 1 teaspoon salt
- 2 eggs, beaten
- 7 or 8 cups flour, enough for soft dough

Soften yeast in 2 cups of warm milk, then add remaining dough ingredients. Let rise double in bulk. Push down and let rise again. This part of the recipe can be done ahead of time and refrigerated, making a separate activity. Frozen dough can also be used.

Shred cabbage and chop onions while meat is browning in skillet. When meat is brown and crumbly, remove from pan. Add enough oil, butter, or margarine to meat drippings to make ½ cup. Place cabbage and onions in the pan and brown, stirring often. Add meat and cover. Simmer for 15 minutes or until cabbage is tender. Cool.

Roll half of the dough at a time to approximately ⅜" thick. Cut into approximately 5" or 6" squares. Place portion of filling in center, then bring corners together and pinch opening securely. Turn pinched side onto generously greased pan or cookie sheet; let rise double in bulk. Bake in a 400°F oven until golden brown, approximately 20 minutes. Makes 24 bunzas. (See a picture of this activity in the opening collage for this chapter.)

Submitted by Christa Yoakum, Program Manager, The Arbors [Memory Care], Madonna Rehabilitation Hospital, Lincoln, NE.

Making Bunzas

Many Germans from Russia settled in Lincoln, Nebraska, in the early 1900s. Their heritage remains important in the community. There are several activities that this community has done to celebrate this heritage, including making cabbage rolls, renamed bunzas. *Persons* with dementia delight in helping with this familiar tradition.

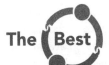

The (Best) Friends Way _____

Life Story: Many *persons* with a German, Czech, or Polish background will recall this dish being made in their home. Others may recall childhood memories of similar dishes. Has anyone had a variation of this dish, such as Argentinean empanadas, Polish pierogi, or British meat pies?

Exercise: Chopping cabbage, stirring the meat mixture, kneading the dough, and filling the bunzas involves both small and large motor skills.

Music: Sing a song in German, such as "Silent Night," or listen to some German music.

Sensory: The meat browning, the cabbage simmering, the yeast bread baking, and the taste of the fresh baked bunzas—all make a sensory feast.

Conversation: Seek an opinion: "Helene, would you taste this for me? Does it have enough salt?" Laugh together: "Heinrich, how many of these could you eat when you were a growing boy?" Reminisce: "Mr. Rhorer, who was the cook in your family?"

Indian Curry

Curried meat and vegetable dishes remain a favorite in many parts of the world, including one of the most populous countries in the world, India. *Persons* with dementia can experience the taste of Indian food, spend time assessing the flavor, and become critics of the taste of curry.

The Basics

Search on the Internet for facts about India and the seasoning curry. India is a fascinating country with many traditions, religions, and diverse landscapes. The use of curry there is traditional.

Curry is a blend of spices. Although recipes differ, ingredients of a curry can include one or more of the following: turmeric, tamarind, coriander, ginger, garlic, chili pepper, cinnamon, cloves, cardamom, cumin, nutmeg, coconut, and even rosewater. The word describes a dish with a sauce. Curries exist in various forms throughout Asia and the world!

Chicken Curry and Tomatoes

4 medium onions, chopped

2 tablespoons curry powder

½ cup butter or cooking oil

1 cup or 1 can (8 ounces) tomato sauce

2 teaspoons salt

1 frying chicken (2 to 3 pounds)

¾ cup hot water

Use a casserole or large skillet with lid. Cook onions and curry powder in butter for 10 to 15 minutes. Add tomato sauce and salt. Cut up and skin chicken; place in sauce. Cook uncovered over medium heat, turning frequently, until sauce becomes quite dry and chicken tests done with a fork. Add hot water, cover pot, and cook over low heat for 5 minutes.

Begin the group discussion with facts about India, including a note about the seasoning of curry. Prepare the recipe for chicken curry and tomatoes, or have it already prepared ready to taste. Serve with basmati rice, a long-grain rice that is used in India, and/or chappatis, a whole-wheat unleavened bread that is fried like a pancake and a standard ingredient of a typical Indian meal. Chappatis may be available in a food shop that specializes in Indian and other ethnic foods or made as a part of the activity.

Submitted by Vinod Srivastava, Family Services, Providence, RI.

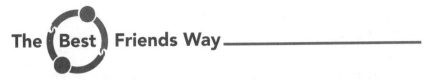

Life Story: Did the *person* enjoy Indian food and occasionally go to Indian restaurants? Does the *person* enjoy eating traditional meat curries such as lamb or beef, or does he or she prefer vegetarian dishes?

The Arts: The Taj Mahal is a landmark of India, and pictures of this beautiful structure can evoke much conversation. Also, Indian saris are beautiful and artfully designed. It would be interesting to have a sari for someone to model.

Music: Listen to recordings of ghazals, a common song form in India today. Ghazals are songs with deep meaning and can be downloaded from the Internet.

Old Skills: Preparing a dish with measuring, stirring, and tasting practices many old skills.

Sensory: The aroma and the taste of curry are very distinctive and stimulating to the senses.

Early Dementia: A *person* could share facts prepared ahead of time on India.

Conversation: Share curiosity: "King, I wonder where curry comes from." Ask for an opinion: "Alma, do you like the taste of curry?" Tie to a life story: "Elizabeth, I understand that the British love their curries. Is that true?" Tease a bit: "Barry, I know you have been a 'globe trotter' and traveled the world. Did you eat local cuisine, or end up at McDonald's?" While serving: "Lulu, do you like your curry with rice or potatoes?"

The Evening Meal

Planning, preparing, and serving the evening meal can be a great time to come together, reminisce, and share about your day. *Persons* with dementia may enjoy participating in aspects of the evening meal, which will help them feel productive and involved.

The Basics

Go above and beyond. Mealtimes for *persons* with dementia should be more than hydration and nutrition; they should be a time for sharing and community. Use activities from this book (e.g., What We Have in Common, p. 35; and Did You Ever?, p. 40) or The Best Friends Way (opposite page) to make mealtime special.

Together, plan your evening meal. For *persons* who still live in their own home, a trip to the grocery store can be pleasurable, particularly if you go during off-hours and keep it short. *Persons* in residential care can participate in some aspect of the evening dinner preparation, including basic meal planning and preparation.

Capitalizing on their strengths, invite the *person* to help you tear the lettuce for salad, chop tomatoes, set the dinner table, stir the batter, or grill the steaks. During the preparation, reminisce with the *person* about his or her evening meals growing up. Before dinner, enjoy a social happy hour (nonalcoholic drinks can be substituted for alcohol) (see Happy Hour, p. 199).

Variation: For the *person* who loves to cook, watch a cooking show or look through food magazines and cookbooks together.

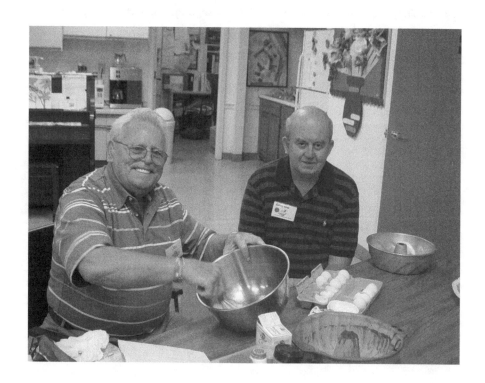

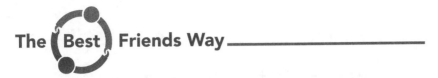

The (Best) Friends Way

Life Story: Who sat together at the evening dinner table? How did the *person* learn to cook? What are his or her favorite foods? Does the *person* have memories of special events, such as Thanksgiving dinner?

Exercise: Preparing the evening meal often involves standing and moving about. This can be especially beneficial and motivating for a *person* who does not move about much during the day. Preparation also may involve chopping, stirring, and shaking, which can be good exercise for eye–hand coordination.

Music: Play soft background music. Break out into spontaneous song or dance in the kitchen!

Humor: Laugh about being famous. Don funny aprons and chef hats.

Old Sayings: "Too many cooks spoil the broth."

Old Skills: Many of the skills that are required for cooking are old skills: e.g., chopping, planning, and stirring.

Sensory: Enjoy all of the stimulating aspects of cooking: the wonderful smells, taste testing, forming meatballs with your hands!

Spirituality: If the *person* prefers, ask a blessing for the meal or invite the *person* to give a favorite blessing.

Early Dementia: Ask the *person* to help plan a menu or share his or her favorite recipe.

Late Dementia: Invite the *person* to sit with you and talk while you do most of the preparations.

Conversation: Ask for advice: "Mom, do you think this dough looks too dry?" Reminisce: "Marion, this potato salad reminds me of your recipe!" Laugh together: "We are covered head to toe in flour!" Share a common favorite: "Lawrence, I can't believe that we both like sushi!" Reminisce: "In our family, when we were children, we all had to stay at the table and listen to the conversation until the grown-ups were finished talking. Lucy, was that the way it was in your family?"

Pie Fest

Homemade pie can conjure up so many memories. For *persons* with dementia, this fun activity about tasting pies evokes old memories, stimulates the taste buds, and celebrates an old culinary tradition.

The Basics

Gather recipes and cookbooks that feature pies and pictures of pies. Discuss pies with the group, including favorite recipes and memories of homemade pies. Discuss the various types of pies, including meat pies (chicken pot pie, shepherd's pie) and fruit pies.

Choose two or three different types of pie to serve to the group: e.g., chocolate, strawberry, pecan, or coconut cream. Pass around the pies for each *person* to assess the appearance. Serve each *person* a small taste of each pie. Invite the group to vote for their favorite pie (see I Cast My Vote For, p. 174).

Variation: Work together to make the pies; debate the dos and don'ts of making the best crusts.

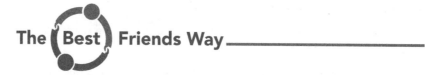

The (Best) Friends Way

Life Story: Does the *person* have a favorite type of pie? Did the *person* enjoy baking? Does he or she have any special tips on the best way to make a good crust? Did the *person* have a sweet tooth? Is there a particular pie associated with the *person's* region, such as Southern Pecan Pie or Oregon Marionberry (a unique Oregon berry with intense blackberry flavor)?

The Arts: Before tasting, hold a contest to judge the "beauty" of each pie.

Exercise: Making pies can be good exercise for the upper body by stirring and rolling the dough or whipping the cream for a topping. Encourage the group to go for a walk after the activity by inviting them to "walk off the calories" from the pies!

Humor: Talk about the comic tradition of getting a pie in your face. Would that still be funny if it happened to you?

Old Sayings: "Four and twenty black birds baked in a pie." "Little Jack Horner." "Pie chest." "Pie safe." "Pizza pies." "Pie in the sky."

Old Skills: Rolling dough, measuring, and following a recipe may be old skills for many.

Sensory: Enjoying food stays with a *person* long into the disease. Savor the pie's aroma and sweet tastes.

Early Dementia: Go to a local restaurant that is famous for its pies for a tasty and fun outing!

Late Dementia: Have a quiet moment and enjoy a sliver of pie together.

Conversation: Ask an opinion: "Do you like fruit pies or chocolate pie best?" Compliment: "Jo Ann, your rhubarb pie is the best I've ever tasted!" Speculate: "What makes a pie a pie?" Reminisce: "What do you think of when I say, 'Coconut pie'?" Learn something new: "Bob, did you ever have shoo-fly pie growing up in the South?"

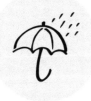

An ounce of prevention . . .

Be aware of persons who have diabetes and be careful not to serve too much sugar.

The Basics _____

Collect some historical facts and trivia about breads, such as the following: The Egyptians were the first to make leavened bread; Krakow, Poland, claims to be the birthplace of the modern-day bagel. Other facts could include varieties of grains used in breadmaking and how breads are made and baked.

Make a list of different and interesting breads, such as corn cakes from Mexico, focaccia from Italy, yeast rolls from the United States, matzo from Israel, pita bread from the Middle East, and baguettes from France. Breads can be made by a group before the session or purchased at a good bread store if you have one in your community. Plan to have one kind of bread baking in a breadmaker timed to be ready to taste during the session.

Talk about bread using some of the facts gleaned from the Internet and books about bread; encourage discussion about the breads liked best or family favorites. Make a list of all of the grains that are used to make bread, such as wheat, millet, barley, rye, rice, corn, and spelt. Pass the breads around for *persons* to see the whole bread. Taste the different varieties with butter added or with flavored olive oils, jams, honey, or cheese if desired.

Variations: Invite a baker to do a "show and tell" demonstration and talk about the different kinds of bread eaten around the world. Make homemade pizzas.

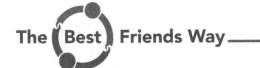

The (Best) Friends Way _____

Life Story: Did anyone grow up in a tradition with a different kind of bread? Who likes sweet cornbread, and who likes cornbread without sugar? Did anyone make homemade bread? Is there an expert on making yeast rolls? Did anyone live in New York City and enjoy frequent meals of bagels and cream cheese (sometimes with grape jelly added!)?

Old Sayings: "Bread of life." "Bread basket of the world." "Bread and butter." "Breadwinner."

Old Skills: Making bread is a skill that is familiar to most *persons*, either doing it themselves or helping with bread making as a child.

Sensory: The aroma from the bread baking is nostalgic and stimulates the appetite.

Early Dementia: Tour a bakery as a group and enjoy samples while socializing.

Conversation: Encourage conversation: "Ginot, did you ever taste bread pudding? In Kentucky, bread pudding is served with bourbon sauce." Ponder: "Marion, I have heard of breadfruit. Is that really bread, or does it just taste like bread?" Confess: "Jake, I like to have bread at every meal. Do you like bread as much as I do?" Discuss: "What is the difference between leavened and unleavened bread?"

Bread of Life

Many cultures and regions in the world have their own version of bread made from many different grains. *Persons* with dementia have grown up with a family favorite or have tried new varieties through the years as they have traveled about or married into a different tradition.

An ounce of prevention . . .

Persons *may be allergic to grains that are used in certain breads.*

Bouquet Garni Herbs

Herbs are known for their many uses, especially flavoring foods. The French use *bouquet garni*, little mixed herb packets that are similar to tea bags, to flavor soups, stews, sauces, and marinades. *Persons* with dementia enjoy making this useful item for everyday cooking.

The Basics

- Fresh-cut herbs, such as basil, parsley, rosemary, and oregano
- Cheesecloth, cut into 4" squares
- Clean, small rubber bands or string long enough to tie a small bundle (5")
- A book about herbs

Use mild fresh herbs such as parsley, basil, thyme, chives, and bay leaves. Different types of recipes call for specific herbs, such as oregano and basil for Italian cooking. Basic cookbooks give an overview of herbs and which foods they flavor best. Try your own blends.

Wash herbs and dry on paper towels ahead of time so that they will be completely dry. Lay out the square of cheesecloth and string. Place herbs in the center of the cheesecloth, then pull up the corners and tie tightly with the string. The planning group (p. 163) can have the herbs washed and dried ahead of time or make a pot of soup using the bouquet garni.

Consider giving the final product a name: "Heritage House Herbs," "Spring Surprise," or "Sunrise Spring Soup Special Herbs."

Tip: Plan to do this activity at a time of year when fresh herbs are easy to come by, such as spring in the Midwest. Make a pot of soup to try out the flavor, then give away the bouquet garni as gifts.

Variations: If you have access to a harvest of lavender, then make sachets (see Making Sachet Bags, p. 213). Make a window garden with a few small herbs in pots so that you always have fresh herbs.

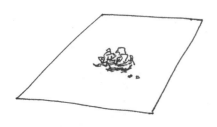

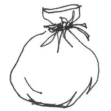

The 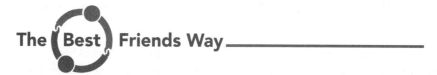 Best Friends Way

Life Story: Know who the cooks and chefs in the group are. What did the *person's* life experiences with herbs consist of (medicinal, culinary, crafts)? Learn about regional uses of herbs. Did someone come from Texas and know just the right way to spice up a barbecue?

Old Skills: Harvesting herbs and cooking are old skills for many.

Sensory: Use herbs with a variety of leaf textures, colors, aromas, and sizes for a pleasing, sensory-rich activity. You can taste a small piece of an herb.

Early Dementia: Explore the folklore of individual herbs and traditional uses.

Late Dementia: Enjoy the unique smells of herbs together by crushing the leaves between your fingers to release the aroma.

Conversation: Ask an open-ended question: "Kathleen, how do you season the stew when you make it?" Ask an opinion: "Aminata, do you like the taste of basil in potato salad?" Reminisce: "Did you ever use fresh mint to flavor your iced teas?" Ask a safe question: "Do you think the word 'bouquet garni' comes from the same place as 'potpourri'?"

The Basics ━━━━━━━━━━━━━━━━━━

Research tasting and share a few facts, such as that our taste buds are found on the tip of the tongue and that the number of taste buds varies, making the way we taste different from one person to another.

    Select a food to be tasted. Examples include white and dark chocolate, varieties of fruit (grapes, melons, and apples are good choices), cookies, cheeses, juices, flavored teas and coffees, and countless other choices. Pass out samples one at a time, and lead a discussion about whether the *persons* like the tastes. Ask *persons* to describe the flavor. Eventually vote on the favorite "temptation" of the day (see I Cast My Vote For, p. 174).

Tip: If several foods are being tasted, then keep the portions to "just a taste."

Variation: Have a wine-tasting party (see Happy Hour, p. 187).

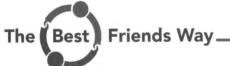

The (Best) Friends Way ━━━━━━━━━━━━━

Life Story: Choose some foods from *persons'* home towns or states to be the focus of the activity, such as cheese from Wisconsin, peaches from Georgia, apples from Washington, wine from California, or clam chowder from New England. Do some *persons* hesitate to taste something new? Who in the group will taste almost anything once?

Music: There may be a song that the *person* associates with the particular food, such as "Don't Sit Under the Apple Tree" or "Picking Up Paw-Paws."

Humor: Laugh about the time we've had to eat a meal even if we didn't like it so as not to offend the hostess.

Old Sayings: "You have good taste." "Good to the last drop" (Maxwell House coffee advertisement).

Old Skills: It is fun to make a dish with a morning group to be tasted later in the day. Many *persons* have old skills that are needed for preparing a dish. Refer to some recipes in this chapter.

Sensory: Tasting can wake up the taste buds and could lead to a full serving for those who liked the taste.

Late Dementia: Tasting can be a joy often to the end of life.

Conversation: Ask for an opinion: "Melissa, did you detect a hint of orange flavor in your muffin?" Agree: "Laura, you are on target. This chili is too spicy." Ask for an opinion: "Margery, does this soup have enough salt?" Tease a bit: "Mike, are you an adventurous eater or a 'meat and potatoes' kind of guy?"

Tempting Tastes

As children, we began deciding whether we liked a food after we dared to taste a bite. Tasting is a great way to get everyone involved without any right or wrong answer, making it perfect for *persons* with dementia.

An ounce of prevention . . .

Check carefully for dietary restrictions.

An Old-Fashioned Tea

Many people have collected teacups, teapots, and fine china, including bone china, English Wedgwood or Royal Doulton, French Limoges, Japanese Noritake, or American Lenox. This activity celebrates the beauty and the history of teacups and pots while providing the *person* with the social engagement of a tea party.

The Basics

Research information on china teacups and tea services. Collect a variety of china teapots and teacups with saucers. Invite families to donate one or two teacups. Have the table set with one or two teapots and a cup and saucer for each *person*. Serve different flavors of tea, and offer cookies or finger sandwiches.

Take the opportunity to evoke old social graces, perhaps finding hats for the ladies and using a tablecloth or some decorative napkins. Encourage conversation and reminiscing, and take in the sensory smell of the tea or coffee.

Variations: Plan a tea party for staff and families. Encourage one *person* to be that day's host/hostess. For more information on tea, see Volume One (Tea Time, p. 184). The group can also discuss the various patterns and styles of china (from modern to traditional) and vote on their favorites. (See I Cast My Vote For . . . , p. 174.)

Submitted by Theresa Nielsen, Activity Director, Alexander Mercy, Royal Oak, MI.

The 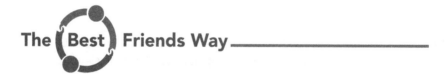 Best Friends Way

Life Story: Is the *person* a tea drinker or a coffee drinker? Did the *person* collect china? Did he or she ever have afternoon tea at a famous hotel in a big city?

The Arts: Study the size and shapes of the cups and pots and the beauty of the intricate designs.

Humor: Joke about holding your "pinkie" finger just right when you sip your tea.

Old Sayings: "Tea time." "Tea for Two and Two for Tea."

Old Skills: Preparing tea and participating in a social gathering may tap into old skills.

Sensory: The warm steam of the tea with the cold feel of the china is a sensory-rich experience. On a nice day, move the activity out-of-doors to soak in the best of nature.

Late Dementia: Enjoy the sensory experience of smelling various herbal teas.

Conversation: Give a choice: "Do you like your tea with milk or sugar?" Debate: "Paula, do men like to drink afternoon tea as much as women?" Ask for information: "Why is it called china? Bone china?" Find a preference: "Mike, do you like sandwiches with the crusts still on or sandwiches without crusts?"

The Basics _____

- Pumpkin seeds from a carved pumpkin (it is okay to include pulp)
- Salt
- Sheet pan for roasting
- Foil
- Nonstick spray
- Large bowls
- Slotted spoons
- Newspaper

Spread the newspaper on the tables to keep them clean while working. Cover the large sheet pan with foil, then lightly spray with nonstick spray. Put the seeds in the bowls and separate from the pulp by filling the bowl with water. Stir the mixture, and the seeds should float to the top.

Remove the seeds with the slotted spoons, stirring as necessary to release more seeds. Continue until most seeds are separated and removed from the bowl. Place seeds on the pan and sprinkle with salt. Bake in the oven at 300°F for 30 to 40 minutes until roasted. Let cool, then serve. Snack on the pumpkin seeds (unlike many seeds, you can eat the whole thing!), and ask everyone present whether they like them.

Submitted by Anne McAfee, Director of Risk Management, Elmcroft Assisted Living, Louisville, KY.

Variations: Roasting sunflower seeds is fun and easy. Soak seeds in salty water overnight. Drain and bake at 300°F for 30 minutes. Another variation is to add sugar and cinnamon for a sweet treat.

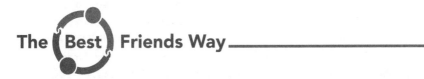

The (Best) Friends Way _____

Life Story: Compare *persons'* long-term memories of harvest time. Discuss any early memories of carving pumpkins. Does someone have a particular fondness for goods made with pumpkin, such as pumpkin pies or bread? Some *persons* may have a diet that consists of vegetables, fruits, nuts, and seeds.

Exercise: The actions of scooping out the seeds and stirring the bowl are good exercise for the upper body.

Old Sayings: "Waste not, want not."

Old Skills: Baking, washing seeds, salting, and scooping all are old skills for many.

Sensory: A pumpkin is rich in sensory sensation. Pumpkin seeds have a distinct smell. The activity of separating the seeds from the pulp is a wonderful tactile experience.

Spirituality: Discuss the meaning of seeds, new beginnings, and cycles of life.

Conversation: Ask a safe question: "What do you think is the difference between seeds and nuts?" Reminisce: "Carla, did you ever roast pumpkin seeds after carving a jack-o-lantern with your children?" Vote: "Miguel, do you like pumpkin seeds or would you prefer another salty snack, such as potato chips?" Ponder together: "Mary Janet, let's make a list of all of the edible seeds that we can think of."

This activity allows *persons* to participate in a seasonal activity while providing a nutritious and fun snack. *Persons* with dementia will enjoy the varied yet simple tasks that are involved in making a snack from pumpkin seeds.

Crazy for Cookbooks

How many of us have dozens of cookbooks that we have collected over the years? Some of them gather dust, but many are in regular use. *Persons* with dementia enjoy a program that is devoted to cookbooks because it evokes old skills and days with family.

The Basics

Obtain 10 or 20 cookbooks from a used bookstore, collections from staff, or donations from residents or family members who no longer use them. Food and recipe magazines can also be collected. Make sure to choose books or magazines with great pictures of the foods. Give everyone a book at which to look. Encourage everyone to leaf through the books. Take one or two special books and read some of the key recipes aloud. Show off any oversized pictures that some cookbooks may feature.

As you pass around the cookbooks, reminisce about favorite recipes or secrets for making familiar dishes, such as meatloaf. Discuss how to plan a dinner party or make a quick snack. Discuss favorite foods; the topics for this activity are endless. It also is a good activity to do before a meal because it will whet everyone's appetite!

Variations: Combine this with a cooking class or demonstration. Pick themes around ethnic food. Make a cookbook of favorite recipes from the group! Pick recipes to cook as a group either immediately following the cookbook discussion or the next day.

The (Best) Friends Way

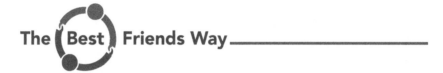

Life Story: Use cookbooks that highlight a *person's* preferred type of food or ethnic or regional background. Was the *person* a collector of cookbooks? What are the *person's* memories regarding cookbooks in his or her family? Did anyone in the group enjoy more exotic ethnic cooking versus American standards, such as meatloaf? Work with families or the *person* to identify and share his or her favorite recipes with the group.

Exercise: Handling the books is gentle exercise for the muscles.

Humor: The subject lends itself to memories of failed soufflés or restaurant meals that did not turn out well. Purchase a big white chef's hat to wear for the program!

Old Sayings: "Too many cooks spoil the broth."

Sensory: The food pictures in the cookbooks may help stimulate appetite.

Early Dementia: *Persons* may enjoy consulting with the chef to plan a menu and/or watch food shows on television.

Late Dementia: *Persons* will enjoy being with others.

Conversation: Make a connection: "Paul, I hear that you are a great cook. It's nice to find another guy who likes to make a good meal for others." Reminisce: "Jeanne, did you enjoy Julia Child, the famous cook on television who introduced America to French cooking? She was really something." Reminisce: "Becky, did you receive a *Better Homes & Gardens* cookbook when you got married?"

The Basics _____

Obtain for this activity:
- Pictures of bees
- Two kinds of honey (one with the comb and one that is strained or two different flavors, such as clover and orange blossom)
- Biscuits and butter (the biscuits can be made earlier in a separate project or be bought)

Before the session, learn all you can about bees and beekeeping, the different kinds of honey, and the various ways in which honey is used. Search on the Internet using keywords: bees, beekeeping, and honey. From the information you have found, prepare several cards of information and trivia that can be read later by *persons* or by the activity leader.

Discuss the information and encourage participation. Look at pictures of bees and talk about any experiences of the group with bees or beekeeping.

Finish the session by tasting the two kinds of honey on buttered biscuit halves. Discuss the kind of honey that is liked better.

Variation: Bake or taste baklava, a Greek sweet that is made with honey.

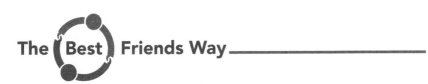

The (Best) Friends Way _____

Life Story: Who may have grown up with hives of bees? Did someone always have honey on the table? Who knows the difference between a honeybee and a bumblebee? Did anyone ever get stung by a bee? Did anyone ever find honey in an old tree or see a swarm of bees?

The Arts: Think of all of the sayings that use the word *bee*, and make a collage of the sayings. Read or recall the story of *Winnie the Pooh* and how the bear stuck his nose in the beehive.

Old Sayings: "Beehive hairdo." "Sweet as honey." "Biscuits and honey." "Busy as a bee." "Queen bee."

Sensory: The aroma and the taste of biscuits and honey are very pleasing.

Early Dementia: *Persons* may respond in a positive way if asked to read the statements about bees and honey.

Late Dementia: *Persons* may enjoy tasting the biscuit and honey.

Conversation: Seek information: "Mr. Paulsell, you said that your family kept bees. Did the bees help pollinate your crops?" Ask an opinion: "Minot, can you tell the difference between this clover honey and this apple blossom honey?" Encourage conversation: "Sara Mae, what kind of flowers do you think bees like best?"

Sweet as Honey

Honey is a staple worldwide and is prized as a special treat in some countries. *Persons* with dementia have enjoyed honey and are fascinated to learn more about this ancient food, a gift from bees and beekeepers.

**An ounce
of prevention . . .**

Note whether anyone is allergic to honey.

Homemade Ice Cream

Many summer picnics and social gatherings are celebrated with homemade ice cream. This activity will provide many memories of good times for *persons* with dementia.

The Basics

Materials/ingredients for each batch (serves 3–4):

- Sealable plastic bags, two sizes: gallon and quart
- ¾ cup milk
- ½ cup half and half cream
- 2 to 3 tablespoons sugar
- Vanilla extract, fresh peaches, bananas, and chocolate syrup
- 3 tablespoons rock salt
- 2½ cups ice

In the small bag, mix the milk, half and half, sugar, and flavors. Place the small bag into the larger bag. Inside the larger bag, add the ice and rock salt so that it surrounds the smaller bag. Release any air that may be inside the larger bag. Make sure that both bags are sealed securely. Shake for 6 to 10 minutes until ice cream is frozen.

After the ice cream is made, invite everyone to taste. While tasting, discuss memories of ice cream.

Tip: Ice cream cones make a good afternoon treat and can calm anxiety and evoke pleasant feelings of childhood.

Variations: Consider making ice cream using coffee cans instead of bags, and roll the cans back and forth. Use an old-fashioned hand-crank ice cream maker (see picture below), but decide on the ingredients as a group.

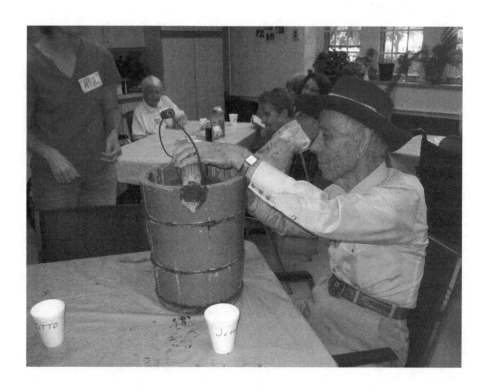

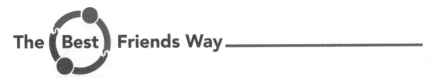

Life Story: Has the *person* made homemade ice cream before? What is the *person's* favorite flavor of ice cream? Did anyone use a hand-crank ice cream maker? Does anyone remember when Baskin-Robbins began with its 31 flavors or recall a favorite childhood ice cream parlor?

The Arts: Make up new combinations of flavors, such as mango banana.

Music: Shake the bags to keep time to an upbeat song.

Exercise: Shaking the bags is great exercise for the arms!

Humor: Have fun: "This better be good for all the work it's taking!" Have a friendly debate about whether homemade is better than store bought.

Old Sayings: "I scream, you scream, we all scream for ice cream."

Old Skills: Preparing food from a recipe is an old skill for many *persons*.

Sensory: The cold feel of the ice coupled with the flavor of the ice cream is a rich sensory experience.

Early Dementia: Visit a local ice cream parlor to enjoy an ice cream.

Late Dementia: A *person* may enjoy observing the process of making the ice cream and reminiscing with others. Choosing the flavor and tasting the ice cream are wonderful ways to participate in this activity.

Conversation: Ask an opinion: "Do you think this is sweet enough?" Encourage participation: "My arm is tired. Would you help me by shaking this bag for a minute?" Reminisce: "Did you ever make homemade ice cream?" Touch the heart: "What do you think about when you think about an ice cream cone?" (childhood, happy times)

**An ounce
of prevention . . .**

Watch for too much sugar intake. Consider substituting Splenda for the sugar for persons who have diabetes.

Hungarian Pogacsa

Every culture has its favorite foods that are made for special occasions. *Persons* with dementia, especially those who are familiar with pogacsa (cheese biscuits), will enjoy making, eating, and even reminiscing about this ethnic treat.

The Basics

The following is a simple recipe from Hungary for pogacsa, made for special occasions such as harvest at summer, grape gathering in the fall, or family gatherings. Pogacsa resembles little cheese biscuits and are especially delicious served warm. See a picture of residents of Zardakert (care home) in Dabas, Hungary, making pogacsa in the picture collage that introduces this chapter.

- 3 packages dried yeast
- ¼ cup warm milk
- 1 pound margarine
- 8½ cups regular flour
- 2 tablespoons salt (or less)
- 3 eggs
- 4 cups sour cream
- ½ pound shredded cheese

Dissolve the yeast in the warm milk and let stand for a few minutes. Mix the margarine with the flour and salt, then add the eggs, sour cream, and yeast mixture. Knead the dough until it is completely mixed. Roll it out to about ¾" thick (approximately as thick as your finger). Cut out the biscuits with a very small cookie cutter. Brush the top of each biscuit with egg yolk and add shredded cheese. Let the pogacsa rise for 1 hour, then bake at 400°F until lightly brown.

Tip: The recipe makes 48 small pogacsas and can easily be reduced or expanded, depending on the number of hungry mouths!

Submitted by Ani Zsolnai, Activity Manager, Zardakert, Dabas, Hungary.

The 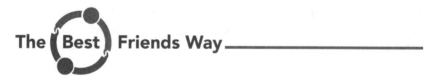 Friends Way

Life Story: Did anyone work in a bakery? Who in the group can share a similar recipe from his or her country? Did anyone grow up in eastern Europe? Who likes to have bread with every meal?

The Arts: Collect pictures of making pogacsa or other baking adventures for all to view and enjoy.

Music: Hum a familiar tune while working together, or enjoy background music.

Exercise: Mixing, stirring, and kneading strengthen the hands and arms.

Sensory: Enjoy the feel of the dough, the aroma of the pogacsa being baked, the delicious taste, and the sights and sounds of laughter as friends work together. Making pogacsa is a sensory feast.

Conversation: Compliment: "Margit, I like the way you make very small, bite-size pogacsa. Is this the way your mother made her pogacsa?" Encourage conversation: "Imre, do these biscuits taste the way your mother made her pogacsa?" Ask for help: "Erzsi, feel this dough. Do you think it needs more flour?" Laugh together: "Vera, don't tell anyone how many biscuits I have eaten!"

CHAPTER NINE

Games and Active Things to Do Together

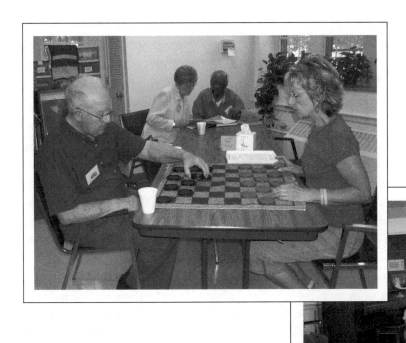

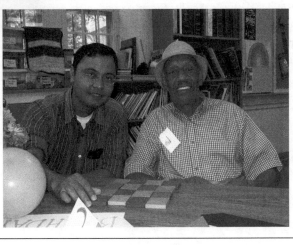

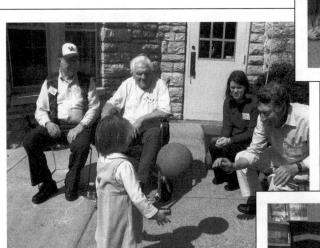

Games and Active Things to Do Together

Almost all of us play games at some point in our life, as children or throughout adulthood. Games can be solitary (e.g., solitaire, video game) or played with other people. They provide valuable socialization, sharpen us mentally, and sometimes provide valuable physical activity. As Shirl Garnett, a *person* with early dementia, shared in Chapter 1, "Games get me thinking and help my spatial concepts, numbers, spelling, and speed of decision."

More and more researchers are suggesting that remaining cognitively active is good for brain health. The saying "use it or lose it" may have more power than we once suspected for all of us.

For *persons* with dementia, games also evoke memories of childhood. In a dementia care program, a fun game or group activity is also a chance for *persons* to "let their hair down," to be a bit silly and have some fun. *Persons* respond positively when their caregivers don't take themselves too seriously—it levels the playing field, so to speak. The best dementia care programs and best caregivers with knack have this friendly "give and take" that the activities in this chapter encourage.

The games in this section include specific games as well as less structured things to do together. They all have been adapted for *persons* with dementia. Specifically, a number of games take advantage of remaining skills that many *persons* have, including

- Retained long-term memories: Long-term memories often remain intact well into a *person's* dementia. Even a *person* who is quite forgetful often remembers and enjoys discussing the meaning of old sayings, such as "Waste not, want not" or "You can lead a horse to water, but you can't make it drink."

- Remaining conversational skills: A *person* may not recognize a picture of a famous individual (e.g., Marilyn Monroe) but might still enjoy discussing her appearance, her outfit, her smile, or even the setting of the photograph if it is apparent (e.g., on the beach, on a movie set). Once the *person* is cued that the individual is Marilyn Monroe, more memories may be recalled.

- Retained physical skills: Some games in this chapter involve physical skills that remain for many *persons*, including good eye–hand coordination.

- Familiar vocabulary: *Persons* often are able to continue spelling words or playing word games. These games seem to rely on deeply learned language skills and rote memories that remain, particularly with some cuing.

We draw your attention to a few specific activities in this chapter:

A number of games that are featured in this chapter are traditional games, some of which may already be part of your activity program. They include Bull's-Eye (p. 164), Bocce Ball (p. 165), and Giant Crossword Puzzle (p. 172). This chapter suggests ways to do these activities with more pizzazz!

Other activities in this chapter involve "things to do together." The activity Fun with Scarves (p. 171) can be a fun one to do at a staff meeting or staff in-service training to encourage staff to "make something out of nothing." County Fair (p. 167) involves more planning but can be an outstanding way to decorate a space and re-create a happy time for *persons,* staff, and families in your program.

Leaf Polishing (p. 179) is a simple activity that *persons* with an interest in plants will very much enjoy. It can be done in the evening or in quiet times or be made into more of a group project.

As we all get older, sometimes the sense of fun and play is lost. Use this chapter as a way of inspiring your inner child. Let loose, and have some fun today!

Tips for staff training: Many effective trainers begin a class with an "ice breaker," or short exercise or game, to warm up the audience and make a point about the learning to follow. Introduce the activities in this chapter by picking one to do together. It makes for a spirited in-service session and can help teach staff how to lead an activity effectively for *persons* with dementia. It can also be effective to ask staff which games they enjoy playing. If someone answers "poker," then you can ask him or her what he or she enjoys about it (e.g., competition, camaraderie, the snacks you eat during the game). Note that *persons* with dementia can experience the same feelings.

CHAPTER NINE ACTIVITIES

The Basics

Select a group of three to five *persons* who are named as helpers or "assistants" to the program leader. Give the group a name, such as Hannah's Helpers, Polly's Planners, or Alex's Assistants.

The group should meet well before the planned group activity. The list of things that may need to be done before the next activity may include arranging tables and chairs to suit the group; getting all of the materials in good order, such as checking the glue bottles and magic markers, sharpening the pencils, sorting materials, and any pre-measuring, cutting, folding, or stapling; or cooking and baking to be tasted later. The group could also do a test run to have a better idea of the needs of the group program, or make samples and patterns for guides—anything to make the group time together more fulfilling.

Be sure to choose occasions to introduce the group to others and publicly thank them for their hard work! Consider an occasional outing for the group to a restaurant or a place for dessert and coffee to thank them for their hard work.

Tip: It is good to have the group meet on a regular basis. There are always things to be done.

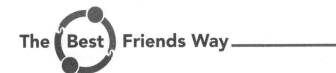

The (Best) Friends Way

Life Story: *Persons* may be chosen to join the group if their life story matches some of the work that needs to be done in the planning session. A builder may be glad to help put together a bird house to be painted later, or a gardener may enjoy gathering flowers to be pressed.

Music: Whistle or hum while you work.

Exercise: Varying levels of exercise are possible, depending on the project.

Humor: Laugh and kid about working too hard or needing a raise in pay.

Old Sayings: "Are we having fun yet?" "Another day, another dollar."

Old Skills: This is a great way to include *persons* with specific old skills.

Sensory: Each meeting may be closed with dessert and coffee, with time to savor the taste of the treat.

Early Dementia: This activity helps a *person* feel needed and productive because he or she can help brainstorm new program ideas.

Conversation: Share a work ethic: "Celia, you and I are just alike. We like to stay busy all day and then fall into bed." Compliment: "Roberta, I like the way you tidy up the lounge. You know how to add that special touch." Reminisce: "Masaka, did your family stay up late at night?" Learn from each other: "Jonesy, I'm learning a new way to keep paintbrushes from getting stiff."

An ounce of prevention . . .

Rotate members of the planning group so that as many persons as possible can participate. This also means that as a person's dementia progresses and he or she is no longer able to participate, he or she will not feel singled out to be dropped from the group.

Bull's-Eye

Maintaining physical activity is very important for everyone. Velcro darts, which can be played inside or outdoors, is a fun way for the *person* with dementia to exercise his or her arms and engage in a healthy competition!

The Basics

Many Velcro dart games are available for purchase at game stores or through activity catalogs.

Set up your Velcro target at an appropriate distance (not too far but not too close to take away the challenge). Take turns throwing the Velcro darts and see who gets closest to the bull's eye. This activity can be done standing or sitting, making it an excellent activity for *persons* with limited mobility. Play as teams and give yourself creative names, such as "The Strong Arms" and "The Dead Shots."

Discuss the history of the bull's-eye and of Velcro. The hook-and-loop fastener was invented in 1948 by Georges de Mestral, a Swiss engineer. The idea came to him after he took a close look at the burdock seeds that kept sticking to his clothes and his dog's fur on their daily walk in the Alps.

Variation: This game can also be played with tennis balls, which also stick to the Velcro target.

The (Best) Friends Way

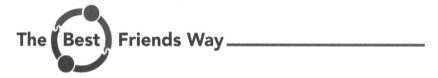

Life Story: Has the *person* played darts in a British pub? Does the *person* enjoy sports? Has he or she always been very active? Is he or she a tennis player? Is he or she competitive naturally?

The Arts: Decorate the target bull's-eye.

Music: Play fanciful music during the game, such as John Philip Sousa's marches.

Exercise: Throwing the darts is great exercise for the upper arms.

Humor: Use self-deprecating humor: "I couldn't hit that bull's-eye if it were the size of my house!"

Old Sayings: "Right on target." "Hitting the bull's-eye."

Old Skills: Playing darts may be an old skill for some.

Sensory: The sound of the Velcro when the darts are removed can be stimulating. Dart throwers might enjoy some snacks while competing.

Early Dementia: If the *person* enjoys darts, encourage him or her to join a dart league in the community.

Late Dementia: Gather *persons* in late dementia close enough to see the movement and feel the excitement.

Conversation: Ask for instruction: "John, show me how you throw those darts. Your technique is so good!" Encourage: "That was so close! You are good at this!" Contemplate: "I wonder why it's called 'bull's-eye.'" Ask with a chuckle: "Vernon, were you a regular at the pool hall in Oshkosh, Wisconsin?"

The Basics

Order a starter set of bocce balls (BocceBallSets.com). The set comes with eight balls of four colors and a small ball called the pallino, or jack ball. Each of the two bocce balls of the same color have distinctive marking for easy identification.

This game can be played on any outdoor surface, such as grass, dirt, or sand. The playing court can be any size to fit the space available. As few as two *persons* and as many as eight *persons* can play this game. Teams can be formed, or individuals can compete against each other.

Toss a coin to determine the team who throws out the pallino first. This ball needs to be rolled within the prescribed playing field. Next, this same team chooses a member to roll a ball as close to the pallino as possible. Then one *person* from the opposing team rolls a ball to try to be closer to the pallino. An opponent's ball can be knocked out of position. The playing continues until all of the balls have been rolled; the team with the ball nearest the pallino wins. Follow the same rules when playing as individuals.

Tip: It is okay to make up a different set of rules depending on the experience of the *persons* in the group. Have fun with the process and don't worry so much about the results.

The (Best) Friends Way

Life Story: This game originated in Italy. Is anyone of Italian descent? Has anyone visited Italy? Who is competitive? Is there someone who is very active and would welcome an opportunity to participate in an outdoor game? Has anyone played other sports involving balls, such as baseball, basketball, or soccer?

The Arts: This is an excellent time for picture taking. Later, display the pictures on a bulletin board or in the art center for all to view.

Exercise: Being out-of-doors and moving about, tossing a ball, and retrieving the balls all encourage good movement.

Sensory: The balls are heavier than expected. Encourage each *person* to hold a ball and try to guess how much it weighs.

Early Dementia: Research some historical facts about this game and ask a *person* to read some of this information to the group.

Late Dementia: Encourage *persons* who chose not to play to be outside and enjoy the fresh air and sunshine while watching the game.

Conversation: Encourage conversation: "Rick, does this remind you of the game of croquet?" "Did you know, Patrick, that this is one of the oldest sports in history?" Give a pat on the back: "Mr. Fritz, you rolled that ball like a professional." Learn from another: "Valentina, show me how you rolled your ball to make it go so far."

Bocce Ball

Most of us are competitors at heart. *Persons* with dementia often retain a competitive spirit and can enjoy a simplified version of this traditional Italian ball game.

An ounce of prevention . . .

Be careful that the ball is not inadvertently thrown at someone since it is heavy.

Hieroglyphics

Ancient languages fascinate many of us. Using stamps to create hieroglyphics (words in ancient Egyptian symbols) is a simple but sophisticated activity for *persons* with dementia.

The Basics

Order a hieroglyphics kit (a variety of kits can be found on the Web, including ones that are sold by museum shops) that includes an ink pad and rubber stamps as well as an introduction to Egyptian symbols and hieroglyphs, how they correspond to the English language, and how to use them to write words and sentences.

Share some facts about the early Egyptians. Choose one or two symbols to enlarge for easy viewing. Talk about their meaning. Discuss why pictures were used to write words and stories.

Encourage *persons* to experiment with using the stamps, first to enjoy the pictures, and then to use them as creatively as each *person* chooses. Spelling one's name in hieroglyphics is always interesting. Help each *person* as needed.

Variation: Use other kinds of decorative stamps (widely available) with your hieroglyphics.

The 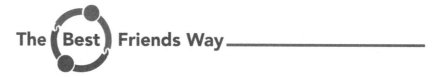 Best Friends Way

Life Story: The *person* may want to spell his or her place of birth, the names of brothers and sisters, or any meaningful person, place, or thing. Who has lived in or visited Egypt? Did anyone see the famous King Tut exhibit when it toured the United States?

The Arts: Each *person's* name, written in hieroglyphics, can be signed, matted, and framed to hang as a colorful display and a conversation piece.

Music: Look for stamps that include musical themes or musical instruments.

Old Sayings: "A picture is worth a thousand words."

Sensory: The feel of the stamp, pressing the stamp onto the ink pad, and viewing the finished product all are very sensory experiences.

Early Dementia: This is an easy activity with lots of history behind it. *Persons* can enjoy reading about the early Egyptians and the development of hieroglyphics in Egypt. When possible, go to a museum if they have antiquities to enjoy.

Late Dementia: With adequate help, a *person* in late dementia may be able to stamp out his or her name.

Conversation: Share a surprise: "Marianne, would you have dreamed that your name would look like this in ancient hieroglyphics?" Wonder together: "Mollie, think how long it would take to write a book using pictures." Reminisce: "Samish, riding that camel by those pyramids must have been quite an adventure. Were you frightened?"

The Basics

Plan to have six to eight booths of interest. Depending on your location, you will know what things are available and of interest. Some ideas are guessing games, such as a big glass bowl full of golf balls to guess the number; a target, such as a hula hoop through which to toss beanbags; some home-canned jars of fruits and vegetables; quilts; cutest baby contest (pictures of babies from which to select); a tasting booth to taste foods such as muffins; and an ice cream booth with places to sit down for an old-fashioned ice cream cone.

Keep the booth displays simple. As an example, at the tasting booth, two kinds of muffins to taste would be sufficient. Prizes can be given at the close of the "fair," and everyone gets a prize for some achievement, whether it be for the one who guessed the right number, or the one who had the most fun, or the one who was the best sport.

Variations: Decorate with bales of hay and bring in a gentle farm animal. Display crafts for sale for a local charity.

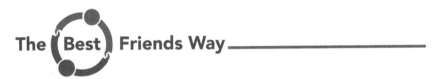

The (Best) Friends Way

Life Story: When planning for this activity, keep in mind the life stories of your group. What interests do you have among your group members? Does anyone have a collection that could make up a booth? Did anyone help with the canning in their early years, or has he or she canned recently? Does anyone have a quilt to add to the collection?

The Arts: You could have a photo booth where the *person* and a friend can have their digital picture made and printed on the spot. Later the pictures can be arranged on poster board, entitled "A Day at the Fair."

Music: Choose lively background music without words. It should set the mood of a fun adventure but not be so loud as to be distracting.

Exercise: This is a good way to get *persons* moving. Before you know it, most *persons* will have moved around a bit without feeling that it was exercise.

Humor: Laugh about adding a kissing booth or when someone wants to skip all except the ice cream booth.

Sensory: The muffins can be made earlier in the day. Just smelling them bake can make the taste buds come alive, and you may have to have one right then and there!

Conversation: Reminisce: "Tony, did you have a county fair in your hometown of Springfield, Missouri, where you grew up?" Encourage: "Ida, let me see you throw this ball right into that hole." Take the blame: "Ivan, I'm sorry I bumped you. Here, try throwing another ring." Share your feelings: "I am really exhausted. Let's sit here."

County Fair

County fairs have been around for a long time and are very much in vogue today. It was a "not to miss" event for many families and provided many memories. *Persons* with dementia can enjoy the re-creation of this popular experience.

Tell Me a Story

Everyone has a story to tell. As we hear a story, it can inform, touch, teach, amuse, entertain, heal, change, or reach the spirit. Stories can give *persons* with dementia many "aha" moments.

The Basics

- Staff or volunteer to lead "story time"
- A quiet area/room with comfortable seating
- A microphone (optional)

Story themes can be on any topic, such as my favorite pet, a holiday, ice cream, vacation, sport, food, and a subject in school. Don't be afraid to try more meaningful topics, including life successes, creative pursuits, work-related achievements, or reflections on historic events (recalling the landing on the moon or the end of World War II). The leader can get the stories started by reading or telling a short story and then asking a question: "Ralph, can you tell me about your favorite hobby?"

The stories can be as brief as a couple of sentences or expanded much longer depending on the *person*. It works well to have the stories at a given session on the same subject, because *persons* will pick up cues from the stories of others as reminders of their experiences.

A roving microphone can be fun for the "ham" storytellers to make the stories seem very important. It is also helpful to be able to hear everyone easily.

Variation: The series of *Chicken Soup for the Soul* books may also prompt discussions with short stories read aloud.

Submitted by Cherry Liter, ACC, a storyteller, Lexington, KY. Resources: National Storytelling Network (www.storynet.org) and International Storytelling Center (www.storytellingcenter.net).

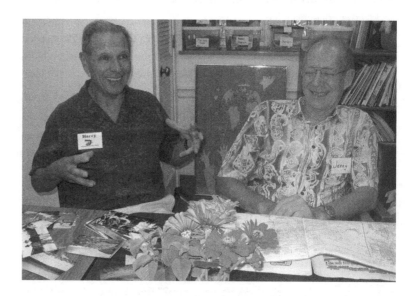

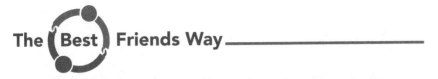
Life Story:　Select storytelling themes that will be familiar to many *persons* in the group. If you know a good story that a *person* likes to share, then build the theme for the day around that story (e.g., vacations in Hawaii). After the story is told, let others tell similar experiences, or ask questions, such as "Have you ever baked a cake that was a disaster?" This activity is a great way to add interesting facts to a *person's* life story.

The Arts:　Record stories for a booklet to give as a gift or to reread later.

Old Skills:　Most everyone has been a storyteller either professionally or as a part of daily life.

Sensory:　Stories can be told in different voices, loudness, and expressions, adding sensory interest.

Early Dementia:　*Persons* may enjoy "journaling" (see Journaling, p. 28) and sharing portions of the stories with the group. One-to-one, they may want to talk about weighty subjects, such as reflecting on their life or relationships with families.

Late Dementia:　If a *person* can no longer tell a story, then he or she may respond to stories by others by a nod or a smile and feel a part of the group.

Conversation:　Ask for help: "Bertha, will you tell us a story about making that red velvet cake?" Encourage participation: "Marvin, you have a great story about meeting a bear in Yellowstone National Park. We would like to hear that story." Compliment: "Ramona, I love your stories." Encourage participation: "Marty, you've had such an interesting life. Tell us about the time you played golf with President Ford."

**An ounce
of prevention . . .**

*Avoid topics for storytelling
that may cause undue
anxiety or sadness.*

The Price Is Right

Over the years, things continue to change, especially the price of everything. *Persons* with dementia may enjoy reminiscing at how inexpensive things were years ago with this fun game.

The Basics

The classic game show "The Price Is Right" is adapted in this activity to create a nostalgic and friendly activity. To prepare, research prices from earlier times, such as the 1920s or 1950s, and take note of prices from today. Gather items to use as props, such as a loaf of bread, a pair of shoes, a purse, a portable radio, or a frying pan, or pictures of larger items, such as a car, washing machine, television set, or pool table. To play, divide your group into two teams. Display the objects. Taking turns, invite each team to guess what the price of the item was in 1950 or whichever year you choose. The team that gets the closest to the price receives 1 point.

The 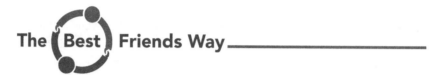 Friends Way

Life Story: Does the *person* enjoy watching game shows? Was the *person* responsible for all of the shopping? Did the *person* ever work in a store? What is the *person's* attitude and values regarding money?

Music: Download music from the game show or some other fun theme song to play during the activity. Sing "How much is that doggie in the window?"

Exercise: Encourage *persons* to move about by inviting them to help you turn over the price cards for the group.

Humor: "I wouldn't pay 2 cents for that old thing!"

Old Sayings: "A penny saved is a penny earned." "Cheap as dirt." "Time is money." "Money is no object."

Old Skills: Social interaction and competition are old skills.

Sensory: To stimulate the senses, encourage *persons* to look at all of the items and explore them before deciding on the price.

Early Dementia: Have the *person* assist you in creating the game.

Late Dementia: *Persons* may enjoy being part of a team and observing and hearing the laughter and fun around them.

Conversation: Seek out attitudes: "Mrs. Swerdlow, do you wait for something to go on sale, or do you buy something when you want it?" Contemplate: "Hugh, do you think $5 for a fancy loaf of bread is too much or just right?" Reminisce: "Rich, what did you pay for your first car?" Ask an easy question: "Sherri, do you enjoy going out to eat at a fancy restaurant now and then, or do you prefer to save money and eat at McDonald's?"

The Basics

Gather an assortment of scarves, including silk, wool, cotton, and nylon, in as many different sizes, shapes, and themes as possible. Large red and blue work "kerchiefs" can also be added to the collection. Brainstorm all of the ways in which scarves can be worn, such as around the neck, over the head, around the shoulders, and around the waist. Experiment with tying a scarf in different ways. Go to the Internet for creative ways to tie a scarf.

Pass out the scarves and enjoy all of the colors and designs. Let each *person* experiment with a scarf. Discuss ways to wear a scarf and have *persons* demonstrate various ways to wear or tie a scarf. The leader might demonstrate scarves being used in other ways, such as keeping time to music, dancing with scarves, making into a halter top, using as a rescue flag, making a scarf chain, using as a way to carry any number of things, designing a bikini, or using as a blindfold. Encourage other suggestions. Discuss each new way in which the scarves can be used.

Fun with Scarves

Scarves come in many sizes, shapes, and colors and can be used for many different purposes. Everyone has owned a scarf or a big handkerchief at one time or another, so *persons* with dementia enjoy this active and sensory activity.

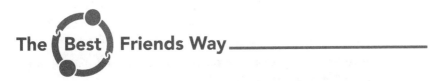

The (Best) Friends Way

Life Story: There may be a *person* who worked in a clothing store where scarves were sold or a *person* who loves to wear all kinds of scarves. Some *persons* may have a fond memory of the big blue and red work handkerchiefs or the big heavy winter wool scarves. Did anyone knit scarves and give as gifts for family or friends? Did she find her scarves on the sale rack for $10 or buy fancy French designer scarves?

The Arts: Tie each *person's* scarf to another until all scarves are together in a long chain. Hang it up for a decorative piece.

Music: Dance while pretending that the scarf is a dancing partner, or keep time with the music while waving a colorful scarf.

Exercise: Exercise with scarves, waving them to the music.

Old Skill: Tying a scarf in various designs is an old skill that is practiced by many.

Sensory: Examine the different designs and themes of the scarves. Feel a cashmere scarf or other soft fabric.

Spirituality: Discuss the religious meaning of covering the head with a scarf before entering a mosque or other places of worship.

Conversation: Recall childhood days: "Beulah, did you always have to wear a scarf around your neck to keep warm during the winters in Montana?" Recall a special trip: "Alvin, that scarf looks like a Scottish plaid and reminds me of your many visits to Scotland." Explore together: "Yolanda, look at this scarf. It has lots of little horses and riders in fancy silks. Let's see if we can count them all."

Giant Crossword Puzzle

Many people have enjoyed working crossword puzzles. *Persons* with dementia, especially those with past experience, can enjoy an adapted version of a crossword puzzle, particularly when the puzzle is done as a group activity.

The Basics

- Large white sheets of poster board
- Magic markers
- Book of easy crossword puzzles
- Easel

Use ready-made crossword puzzles or create your own. Puzzles that have a theme or particular subject, such as summertime or everything about dogs, are particularly effective. Re-create the blank crossword puzzle on the poster board. Go to the Internet for ready-made puzzles.

Discuss the nature of the puzzle, then begin by giving a clue, such as, "One down is a five-letter word for a young dog." The leader might repeat by saying, "What is a five-letter word for a young dog?" As an answer is given, try to fit it into the spaces. Keep giving opportunities to give the right answer, and if no one comes up with it, you may say, "What about the word 'puppy'?"

Tip: Take time to discuss the answers, because this adds extra interest and cognitive stimulation to the activity. Continue until the puzzle is finished or you decide to finish it another time.

Variation: Use 8 to 10 facts from a *person's* life to design a crossword puzzle. The answers can be scrambled at the bottom of each puzzle. Also, the format can be changed to "fill in the blanks."

Submitted by Nancy Kahler, Certified Nursing Assistant/Activities, Sentry Hill at York Harbor, York, ME.

The 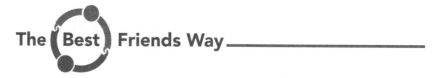 Best Friends Way

Life Story: When possible, incorporate everyone's life story in some way. Each clue can have numerous possibilities for connections to a *person's* life. If the clue's answer is "poodle," then you can point out that three *persons* in the group have owned poodles. A complete puzzle can be made on the facts of one *person's* life.

Music: One puzzle could be all about music or *persons'* favorite songs or dances.

Old Sayings: Make a puzzle by finishing old sayings, such as "Waste not (want not)" or "Two heads are better than (one)."

Spirituality: Incorporate the name of a *person's* religious ritual or symbol into a puzzle.

Early Dementia: The *person* may enjoy reading out the clues.

Conversation: Be surprised: "Claude, I never knew you played bocce ball in Italy. That was a difficult word to spell out, and you did it." Encourage: "Mimi, you are on the right track. What about trying the word 'chicken' for 8 across?" Have fun: "Rosa, I would rather be eating 'Rocky Road' ice cream than spelling it on this crossword puzzle. Wouldn't you?" Discuss the answers: "The word is 'lasagna.' Did your mother make a good lasagna?"

The Basics _____

Collect 6 to 10 objects for the scavenger hunt. Themes can be chosen, such as kitchen utensils, small musical instruments, balls (e.g., soccer, tennis, footballs), or gifts to be given to the children's hospital. Select a space for the scavenger hunt. Depending on the objects to be hidden and the weather, the hunt can be held inside or outside. The space for searching should be in a definite prescribed area so as not to be too confusing.

Make some things easy to locate and a few articles more difficult. After the items have been found, discuss each one.

Tip: This activity requires additional volunteers to provide cues and prompting during the hunt.

Variation: Plan a holiday scavenger hunt around Easter, Halloween, or Christmas.

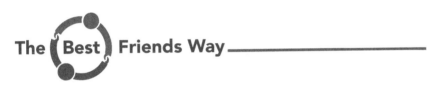

The (Best) Friends Way _____

Life Story: Choose themes to match life stories and connect *persons* with the objects located, such as a football player with the football, a good cook with a muffin pan, or a musician with a tambourine.

Music: If music is the theme, then after all of the instruments have been found, use the instruments to make music.

Exercise: Encourage everyone to participate. Every time *persons* with dementia have a reason to move about, it can be therapeutic.

Humor: Look for things to laugh about: the drum in the tree or the hat on the statue.

Old Sayings: "If it had been a snake, it would have bitten me." "Finders keepers." "Looking for a needle in a haystack."

Old Skills: Looking for hidden or lost articles is an old skill that we all have practiced.

Sensory: After the scavenger hunt, pass around the articles to be examined. The gifts to be given to the children's hospital could also be wrapped for sensory input.

Early Dementia: *Persons* can help with hiding the articles and help keep track of the hunt. They might enjoy tracking down articles that are not easily found by others.

Conversation: Ask for help: "Susan, can you help me find a bread pan?" Laugh: "I spend most of my time looking for things." Ask for an opinion: "Richard, would you like to do a little golf putting now that we have found this ball?" Compliment: "Lavonia, you spotted that bell as quick as a wink."

Scavenger Hunt

A scavenger hunt is reminiscent of intrigue and excitement. When it is redesigned to be appropriate for *persons* with dementia, it can be an activity that caregivers and *persons* both can enjoy.

I Cast My Vote for . . .

Voting is an old skill that touches on civic duty and patriotism. *Persons* with dementia can feel empowered by taking part in simple votes—e.g., for which person, place, or thing that they like best.

The Basics

Collect pictures of the greatest variety of persons, places, and things, such as fashions, houses, babies, animals, flowers, sports, and desserts. Offer two of the same category, then ask questions such as, "Which mustache do you like better?" or "Which baby do you think is cuter?" or "Which chair do you think would be more comfortable?" or "Which man looks happier?"

This can be a one-to-one experience or a group project. In a group, be sure that each *person* has the opportunity to express him- or herself. Record the vote of each *person,* then announce and show the winners at the close of the session.

Variation: Bring in actual objects to vote for as favorites, such as different kinds of purses or different styles of sunglasses. Create paper "ballots" for some activities.

The 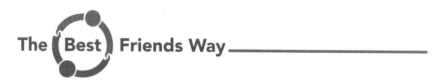 Best Friends Way

Life Story: Pictures can be chosen with the life stories of the group in mind. You may have a sports *person,* a builder, a collector of purses, a proud grandmother, or a lover of animals in the group. If pictures that represent something in the *person's* life story are used, then conversation can continue around the interest. Did the person make it a practice to vote in local, regional, or national elections?

The Arts: Two pictures by famous artists can be presented and discussed before voting for a favorite. Conversation can follow about why a particular picture was chosen. Was it design, color, or characters?

Music: You can listen to two types of music and vote for the one that is liked better.

Sensory: Looking for details and differences in pictures can stimulate the sense of sight.

Old Sayings: "Ballot box." "Election day." "One man (woman), one vote."

Old Skills: Giving preferences is an old skill that has been fine-tuned by years of experience. Many *persons* with dementia can respond to casting a vote.

Spirituality: Use pictures that evoke the spiritual, and ask which picture makes one feel better. Self-esteem results from knowing that your opinion counts.

Early Dementia: This activity can be as complex as you need it to be. It can involve poetry, architecture, literature, sculpture, or current events.

Conversation: Ask for help: "Margaret, I can't decide which necklace is better to wear with this dress. Which necklace do you like better?" Seek an opinion: "Brad, do you think it is good to have a strong opinion about things?" Laugh together: "Do you think either of these outfits is worth our vote?" Encourage an opinion: "Beverly, I'm trying to decide which of these two men in this picture looks happier. What do you think?"

The Basics _____

Search for a car with a sound body. It should have no rust or sharp edges, and a clean, attractive interior—ideally a classic car from the 1940s, 1950s, or 1960s, or a car with some unusual character (a Volkswagen Bug or convertible) is ideal. You may be lucky and have a car donated. Build a storage shed or covered space to house the stationary car; include room for a workbench and storage space for buckets and cleaning supplies. Keep the battery charged so that the radio works. It is helpful to have a comfortable surrounding to encourage socialization for those who want to converse while others work on the car.

Encourage car lovers to spend time working on the car, polishing or waxing, or just sitting in the car and listening to the radio. "Happy hour" or a tailgate party can be enjoyed in this vicinity late in the afternoon (see Happy Hour, p. 187).

Adapted from submission by Patricia Wesley, Administrator, Omanhanui Private Hospital, New Plymouth, New Zealand, in The Best Friends Staff: Building a Culture of Care in Alzheimer's Programs *by Virginia Bell and David Troxel (2001), www.healthpropress.com.*

In My Merry Oldsmobile

What car lover does not like to admire and/or tinker with a classic car? *Persons* with dementia may maintain the love of working on a car and enjoying the shine of a new polish job.

The 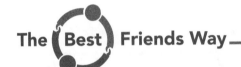 Friends Way _____

Life Story: Which kind of car does the *person* like best? What model or brand was his or her first car? Was he or she the one in the family to take care of the car? Who likes to shop for a car? Did anyone have a convertible? Was anyone a mechanic?

The Arts: Take pictures of *persons* sitting in the car or pictures of *persons* working on the car for a photo display.

Music: Sing or listen to the music "In My Merry Oldsmobile" or "See the USA in a Chevrolet." Find a good music channel on the car radio and listen while socializing.

Exercise: Waxing and polishing the car is good exercise, all in the out-of-doors.

Humor: Encourage this time to be light-hearted and fun. Laugh about what went on in the "rumble seat" or slipping the car out without permission.

Old Sayings: "On the road again."

Old Skills: A good wax job on their favorite car is something that many *persons* have admired many times.

Sensory: The feel of being outside and smelling the cleaning fluids and wax help a *person* recall past routines and chores.

Conversation: Share a story: "Melvin, my family always drove a Buick. Do you like Buicks?" Help a *person* feel important: "Mildred, I love being with you because you have so many interests. You know more about cars than anyone I know." Reminisce: "Carl, did you ever have to change a flat tire?"

Color Wheel

Games such as "Wheel of Fortune" and "Jeopardy" have been in our homes for years. *Persons* with dementia, like all of us, have entered into the spirit of these games. This activity is a homemade, simplified version of a game show.

The Basics

- Poster board
- Magic markers
- Watercolors
- Paintbrushes

With a black magic marker, draw a circle to fill the poster board and divide the circle into six to eight segments. Using watercolors, paint the segments different colors. Design questions from material that is familiar to *persons,* such as people (U.S. presidents), places (Hollywood), and things (nicknames of the states). The questions should be familiar but difficult enough to be of interest. Develop at least four questions per color.

Divide the group into two teams. Ask a *person* on one team to choose a color, then ask a question that can be answered by anyone on that team. If no one on the team knows the answer, then the question goes to the other team. The second team, however, always gets a turn, even if they have answered the first team's question. Continue until each *person* has chosen a color or until all of the questions have been answered. The activity does not have to be a competition, but you can score the event and give the team that gets the most correct answers a prize (but also have a prize for the second place team!).

The 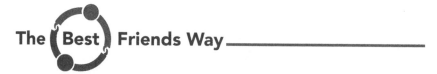 Best Friends Way

Life Story: Use ideas from the life stories to formulate the questions for the game. Examples could include writing questions about baseball trivia for a sports buff, Hollywood trivia for a movie fan, or common herbs for a gourmet cook.

The Arts: *Persons* can be involved in making the color wheel.

Music: Play theme songs from the game shows to begin the game and/or during the game (available from the Internet).

Humor: Choose some humorous questions, such as, "Do you really believe that the cow jumped over the moon?"

Old Skills: Choose names for the two teams. It is an old skill to choose teams and compete against each other.

Late Dementia: Create simpler questions that have no right and wrong answers, such as: "What is your favorite color?" "Do you like peppermint ice cream?" "Do you like to watch football?" "Do you like to go to bed early?" "Do you like to swim?" These questions can help some individuals later in dementia feel successful and a part of this game.

Conversation: Reminisce: "Roberto, I'm not surprised that you were the valedictorian of your class. You have the answers on the tip of your tongue." Ponder: "Margaret, I'm wondering when 'Wheel of Fortune' began. Do you know?" Encourage: "Harry, you have named two of the oceans, the Atlantic and the Pacific. What about the ocean around the North Pole?"

The Basics _____

- Flipchart
- Marker

Select words that are associated with being an adult but are familiar, such as "healthy," "coffee," "language," "content," or "beautiful." Call out the word, offer a simple definition, repeat the word, and ask for volunteers: "Who would like to try spelling 'fragrant'?" If the correct answer is given, then write it in large letters on a flipchart. Let others try if the correct spelling is not given. Give clues or fill in some letters if needed.

Try to include everyone in the conversation, even those who are not attempting to spell. The word may remind you of something in that *person's* experience. Spend time talking about any connections. Continue as long as there is interest in this idea.

Variation: Two spelling groups can be formed to take turns spelling words. Name the groups using creative names, such as Sam's Spellers or Betsy's Bunch.

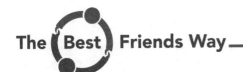

The (Best) Friends Way _____

Life Story: Plan to spell the state or country of birth of each *person*, and spend time talking about his or her birthplace. Spell the months, and note each *person's* birthday. Try to spell each *person's* name. Who remembers spelling bees? Who was a good speller, and who admits that he or she was a miserable speller?

Music: Try to spell "supercalifragilisticexpialidocious," a very long word in a song from the musical "Mary Poppins," and then sing some of the song.

Humor: Have some friendly competition between the two groups. Joke with each other about who is the best at spelling.

Old Skills: The skill of spelling remains intact for many *persons* until late into the disease.

Early Dementia: A *person* could help write the correctly spelled word on the flipchart.

Conversation: Enjoy the time together: "Sam, we are having such a great time trying to spell these words. I can tell that you are having as much fun as I am." Celebrate: "Katrina, you spelled that difficult word. I'm impressed." Prompt with dignity: "Stanley, that is so close. Try a 't' on the end of the word, and I think you will have it correct." Ask for help: "Mrs. Jones, would you help me with my English studies? How do you spell this word?"

Spelling Bee

Spelling bees are something with which we all are familiar. Have you ever asked a *person* with dementia to help you spell a word? You may be surprised at all of the good spellers. A spelling bee lends itself to one-to-one or group environments and is a perfect intergenerational activity.

An ounce of prevention . . .

If someone misspells a word, then you might say, "That's close." Watch for those who may be anxious about trying to spell.

Matching Squares

This activity involves making a puzzle that can be used over and over. *Persons* with dementia can enjoy the making and, later, the reconstruction of a great variety of puzzles.

The Basics

- Discarded wallpaper sample books available from designers or home decorating stores
- Magazines with colorful pictures
- Enlarged photos
- Poster board
- Glue
- Scissors

Choose a 9" × 9" section that contains a design or a picture from any of the above materials. When making your own squares, plan for some with special interest to men, such as military items, farm equipment, or cars. Trim neatly and glue it to a poster board backing. When dry, cut into nine (3" × 3") squares. An assortment of these challenging puzzles can be kept on hand for a "grab and go" activity.

Variations: To purchase nine-piece puzzles, called "Scramble Squares," go to www.b-dazzle.com. You have the choice of more than 100 different squares.

The 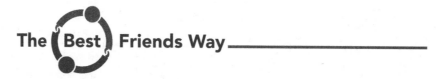 Best Friends Way

Life Story: Each picture or design can have a story. Relate the story to anything in a *person's* life that is familiar. It may be a scene of a lake, a river, or a mountain that is reminiscent of the *person's* childhood locale. With the use of a digital camera and a copier, design pictures to be made into puzzles of *persons* with their friends.

The Arts: Once the pictures of *persons* are reconstructed, they can be reglued on cardboard and arranged as an exhibit for all to enjoy.

Music: Create some squares around musical instruments, song lyrics, or sheet music.

Old Skills: Encourage cutting, pasting, smoothing, and selecting.

Sensory: Note the smell of the paste and reminisce about school days.

Spirituality: The pictures can portray some spiritual moment for the *person*, such as a picture of a sunset, a country church, or a picture of Buddha.

Early Dementia: *Persons* may enjoy the "Scramble Squares" because they tend to be more challenging.

Conversation: Comment on the puzzle once it is put together: "Jack, what do you think these people are doing in this picture?" Share something in common: "Doris, great minds think alike! We both start in the middle of the puzzle and work to the edges." Have fun: "Roger, look at this hairdo. Would you like a haircut like this one?"

The Basics _____

Work with *persons* to gather potted plants that are light enough to be moved. Bring them to a table for easy access for the *persons* to clean and polish the leaves. The larger plants/trees in the decorative pots can be attended by *persons* who have good mobility and balance. Use a product called "leaf shine" or "leaf polish," which is made especially for indoor plants. Spray the plant with the product and encourage the *person* to wipe each leaf, eliminating any dust build-up and producing healthy, shiny leaves.

Submitted by Rosemarie Harris, Director, Pinegrove at Vista del Monte, Santa Barbara, CA.

Variations: Go to a nursery or farmer's market to buy new plants to add to the community collection. Also, consider putting together a community plant sale.

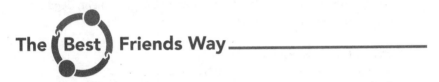

Leaf Polishing

Leaf polishing is an activity that the residents at Pinegrove of Vista del Monte in Santa Barbara, California, enjoy each week. The activity involves *persons* maintaining and enhancing the potted plants in their home.

The (Best) Friends Way _____

Life Story: Does the *person* enjoy plants and gardening? Has the *person* been a good housekeeper? Did the *person* have potted plants at home or at his or her office? Use elements of the life story throughout the activity to have fun visiting and reminiscing during the activity.

The Arts: *Persons* could take one of their favorite plants and sketch it or use it as inspiration in some other art project.

Music: Play fun instrumental background music while polishing.

Exercise: Gathering the plants and polishing the leaves encourage *persons* to move about and stretch their legs and arms.

Humor: Laugh while commenting, "I never thought I would be known as a leaf polisher."

Old Sayings: "A green thumb." "A rose is a rose is a rose."

Old Skills: Tending to one's home is an old skill for many.

Sensory: The colors of the plant leaves and clean smell of the leaf polish can stimulate the senses. Notice the differing shades of green and try to name them.

Early Dementia: *Persons* with early dementia can try to identify and label each plant for future reference.

Late Dementia: Invite the *person* to help you by inspecting your work and making sure that you didn't miss any spots on the leaves.

Conversation: Encourage participation: "Mac, can you help me gather the plants for our leaf polishing?" Compliment: "You are so helpful. Thank you for faithfully cleaning the plants each week." Ponder together: "Cleta, they say you should talk to your plants to make them healthy. What should we say to this hibiscus?"

Decorating Pumpkins

Pumpkins are a staple food used around the world. Carving pumpkins will evoke happy memories for many who did this activity as children or with children and grandchildren.

The Basics

Obtain pumpkins from a store or during an outing to a pumpkin patch. There are three methods of decorating a pumpkin:

Traditional Jack-o-Lantern

- Pumpkins
- Carving knife
- Newspapers
- Marker
- Wooden spoon
- Votive candle

Design and mark the places to be cut on the pumpkin with the marker. Cut out the top around the stem first. Cut at a 45° angle so that the "lid" will not fall in. Remove the seeds and pulp from the inside with a large wooden spoon (see Pumpkin Seed Roasting, p. 153). Cut out the eyes, nose, and mouth for the face. Put a votive candle inside.

Tip: Line the cuts with petroleum jelly so that the pumpkin will last longer.

Submitted by Anne McAfee, Director of Risk Management, Elmcroft Assisted Living, Louisville, KY.

Painted Faces (no cutting)

- Tempera paint
- Paintbrushes
- Newspapers
- Pencil
- Black marker

Draw your design on the pumpkin with a pencil. Go over the pencil marks with the marker so that the lines to be painted will be easily seen. Paint as desired. Allow to dry.

Tip: Paint a coat of shellac over the pumpkin to make it last longer.

Carved Method

- Pumpkin
- Purchased patterns and tool kit (may be purchased at a grocery store)

Prepare the pumpkin by cutting the lid around the stem and cleaning out the seeds and pulp. Use a purchased pattern or draw one on paper freehand. Place the pattern over the pumpkin and tape it down. Poke holes around the designs with a poking tool that comes in the kit, or use a nail. Remove the pattern and cut from hole to hole.

The (Best) Friends Way

Life Story: Notice details about personal interests that might apply to pumpkins, such as favorite color orange, farmers, or cooks. Who grew pumpkins as a family? Does anyone like to eat pumpkins, baked or in pie?

The Arts: Draw new designs for the painted face pumpkins.

Humor: Make a jack-o-lantern with a big winking eye.

Old Sayings: "Peter Peter Pumpkin Eater, had a wife and couldn't keep her, put her in a pumpkin shell, and there he kept her very well."

Sensory: Listen to the sound of your hand gently patting on the pumpkin. Be sure to feel all of the textures of the outside of the pumpkin, the inside, and the stem and what it feels like to carry. Enjoy the smells of traditional pumpkin spices such as nutmeg and cinnamon.

Early Dementia: Encourage the *person* to make design decisions and draw the design on the pumpkin.

Late Dementia: Make eye contact; ask for an opinion about how he or she likes the face on the pumpkin.

Conversation: Ponder: "Jody, I wonder why pumpkins became part of Halloween." Ask a safe question: "Harold, what do you think of when you see a load of pumpkins?" Ask for advice: "Do you think that we should serve whipped cream with the pumpkin pie?" Celebrate the life story: "Yalmin, did you eat pumpkins in season when you were growing up in Istanbul?"

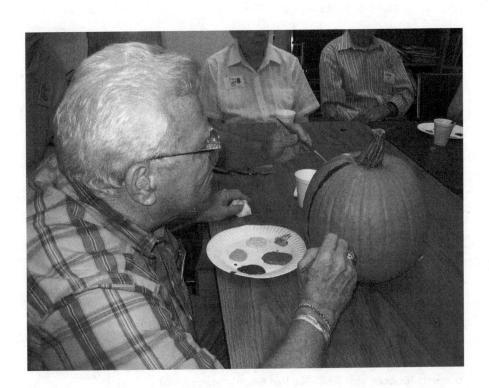

Flannel Boards

Flannel boards are colorful and tactile bases that can be used over and over again for art projects or to tell a story or evoke a theme. *Persons* with dementia may enjoy creating these simple but useful boards for a variety of art projects.

The Basics

- Flannel material for board (yellow works well)
- Pieces of different-colored flannel or felt (may be leftover scraps)
- Thin masonite board
- Poster board
- Material with some body, such as batting
- Scissors
- Tape
- Glue
- Wooden picture framing border, approximately ½" to ¾" wide

The frames can be any size, but 14" × 20" works well for individual flannel boards. These can be made in your program if you have the interest and the equipment. Also, if there is a woodworking shop in your community, they might take on the project and welcome some *persons* from your group. Otherwise, they can be made in a frame shop.

Cut a piece of poster board to fit into the frame. Cut a piece of the batting and a piece of flannel the size of the poster board. Cover the batting with the flannel and staple it to the poster board. Cut the masonite to fit inside the back of the frame. Put the flannel board into the frame, then glue the masonite into the back of the frame.

Cut colored pieces of flannel or felt into shapes or figures. Encourage *persons* to choose pieces and arrange them on the flannel board. This activity is especially effective when children are involved.

Variation: New or old picture frames can be used by cutting the material, posterboard, and masonite board to fit within the frame.

The (Best) Friends Way

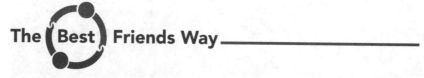

Life Story: Individual designs can be cut to reflect a *person's* interest, such as animals, a canoe and paddle, a cake and a rolling pin, or a football and jersey.

Old Skills: Working with children to help arrange the pieces on the flannel board and then telling the story both are old skills, as is sorting fabric by size and color.

Sensory: The warm feel of flannel can be a reminder of flannel nightgowns, pajamas, and sheets for those who grew up in places with cold winters.

Spirituality: Religious symbols, such as a cross, a star, a candle, or a dove, can be used as felt pieces.

Late Dementia: If someone in your group is very tactile, then arranging and rearranging these pieces can be a source of pleasure in very late dementia.

Conversation: Explore: "David, look how this felt canoe sticks to the flannel board." Encourage: "LaVonne, let's create a quilt square. You can help me." Compliment: "Debbie, that looks like Van Gogh's 'Starry Night.'"

CHAPTER TEN

In the Evening

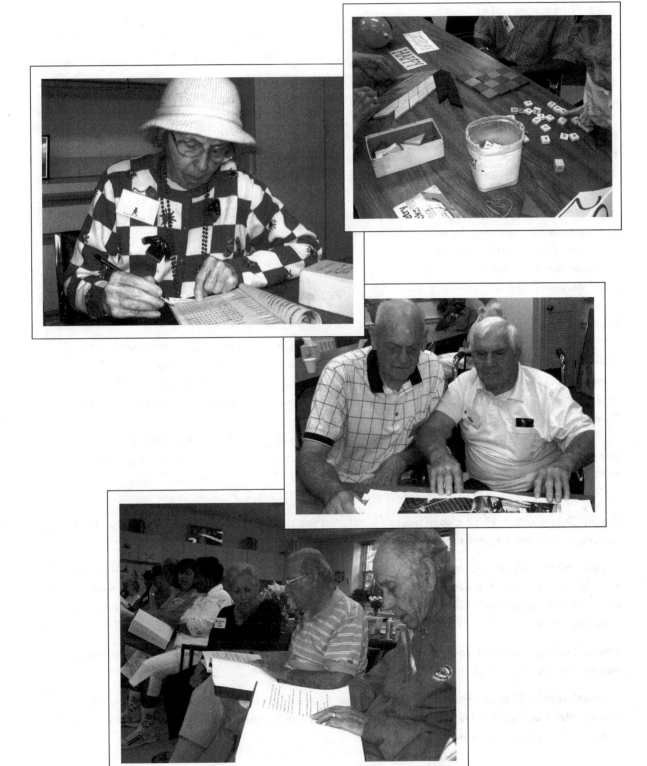

In the Evening

It is disappointing that many otherwise good dementia care programs have so little to offer in terms of activities in the evening. Sometimes *persons* with dementia go to bed early; we understand that sometimes the demands of the day have worn them out. In other cases, we suspect that *persons* are going to bed early out of boredom or lack of stimulation.

Having an evening activity program in a residential facility is a mark of quality and supports dignity and happiness by improving the quality of life. Even small efforts in this area will pay dividends.

Evenings are often a time to wind down, yet for *persons* with dementia, don't make the mistake of assuming that they cannot handle any challenges in the evening or that this might disturb that night's sleep. We believe that a rich evening program does quite the opposite: It supports self-esteem and allows *persons* to turn in feeling more content (and maybe just a bit more tired), thereby facilitating a better night of sleep.

For example, one activity program leader told us that there should be little to no stimulation after dinner—maybe just some quiet music, hand massages with lotion, or reading of a poem. We like those three activities but disagree with her view. We suspect that there are at least some residents who are used to doing more productive and interesting things at night, and we should give them an opportunity to do these things.

Remember that one Best Friends principle is that "if you've met one *person* with Alzheimer's disease, you've met just one *person* with Alzheimer's disease." Some may benefit from a quiet evening, but others need much more.

We draw your attention to a few specific activities in this chapter:

Evening Busy Room (p. 197) is a good place to look for ideas about how to create an activity space for the evening, particularly for *persons* who like to stay up late or who wake up during the night.

Happy Hour (p. 187) can be held once a week or once a day! Build in a happy hour with alcohol-free cocktails (unless the doctor has okayed some wine or beer) to give *persons* something to look forward to before or after dinner. We know that happy hour is usually before dinner, but we think you can bend the rules somewhat!

Playing Cards (p. 189) is the simplest of activities but one that can be meaningful, productive, and important for *persons*.

Johnny Carson (p. 203): Generations of individuals went to bed watching "The Tonight Show" with Johnny Carson. With the advent of DVDs and video, many of his old shows are available. Have a regular "night with Johnny" to cap off the evening.

Many of the activities in this chapter will be valuable for home-based caregivers. For those in long-term care, we encourage you to view your program as a 24-hour day. Try to have options available whatever the hour.

Tips for staff training: A key for this chapter is to challenge many staff members' views that evening programs "will not work." To do this, we encourage program leaders to work an occasional after-dinner shift and bring some activities in this chapter (or others from the book) to demonstrate. When staff members see residents participating, many of their preconceived notions will dissolve.

CHAPTER TEN ACTIVITIES

The Basics _____

Choose a regular gathering place and time for happy hour. Late afternoon, such as 4:00 p.m., may work well and may provide a good distraction from the end-of-the-day concerns. Serve snacks and drinks according to the *person's* preference, and facilitate light conversation. (In some cases, alcohol is appropriate; substitute nonalcoholic beverages such as sparkling cider or nonalcoholic beer when advisable.) Invite those present to make a toast to a special individual or to the group.

Happy Hour

Many of us have enjoyed the ritual of unwinding from the day by celebrating "happy hour," a time for a glass of wine or a cocktail and a snack accompanied by good conversation. At a time of many transitions of the day, *persons* with dementia may enjoy relaxing with friends for conversation and a "cocktail."

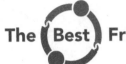

The (Best) Friends Way _____

Life Story: Has the *person* enjoyed parties or happy hour? Did the *person* have a regular before-dinner drink, such as a glass of wine or a martini or a soft drink? Did he or she ever belong to a country club or other clubs with a happy hour? Conversely, did the *person* believe that drinking was not appropriate?

The Arts: Take pictures for a happy hour picture gallery.

Music: Play fun instrumental background music to help set the mood. Invite a musician to entertain the group during happy hour.

Exercise: Hold happy hour on the patio or in the garden in good weather, adding movement for health.

Humor: Invite the joke teller of your group to share a favorite joke. Toast for every occasion, even humorous occasions, such as seeing the resident dog fetch Terry's hat.

Old Skills: Talking, socializing, and entertaining with others help *persons* maintain old social skills. Invite family members or staff occasionally to join the group for a drink.

Sensory: The sights and sounds of a party can be joyous and uplifting for many. Often a drink can stimulate appetite.

Conversation: Celebrate: "Hazel, it is fun to relax with you after we have both had a busy day. What fun to be together." Laugh at the size of the drink: "Raymond, this is real inflation! Look at my tiny glass of wine." Share a joy: "I would like to make a toast to Gladys for her new hairdo. She looks younger than ever!" Rejoice: "Let's raise our glasses to this beautiful day and a restful night's sleep!"

An ounce of prevention . . .

Use common sense when setting limits around alcohol consumption.

Mysterious, Magical Moon

The moon has long been associated with romance and mystery. *Persons* with dementia may enjoy sharing their own opinions, observations, or experiences that are relevant to the moon.

The Basics

Gather up the *Farmer's Almanac* and all of the folktales and moon phase and tide charts that you can find for a friendly discussion about the moon. (For more facts about the moon, go to the following Web sites: www.moonconnection.com and en.wikipedia.org/wiki/Moon.)

Share known facts about the moon, such as that the Apollo missions brought back 2,196 rock samples; there are two places in the world where a moonbow can be seen: Victoria Falls, Africa, and Cumberland Falls, Kentucky; and from the moon, the astronauts could see the Great Wall of China.

If it is a balmy evening, go out and "moon gaze." Otherwise, gather and show pictures of the moon.

The 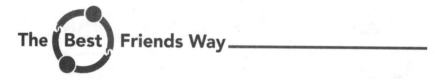 Best Friends Way

Life Story: Did anyone in the group or their parents or grandparents follow the *Old Farmer's Almanac* for moon phases for planting or harvesting? Did the *person's* family celebrate the Lunar New Year (see Lunar New Year, p. 89)? Who in the room recalls how they felt on the day the astronauts landed on the moon?

The Arts: Draw the fictitious man in the moon. Create a collage about space travel, the universe, or astronauts.

Music: Sing a song about the moon: "Shine On, Harvest Moon" or "Moon River."

Humor: Exclaim over the nursery rhyme "Hey diddle diddle, the cat and the fiddle, the cow jumped over the moon."

Old Sayings: "Silvery moon." "Moon Pie." "Blue moon" (second full moon in 1 month).

Sensory: Seeing the moon shine brightly on a warm summer evening is a chance to go outside. Enjoy a moon-pie snack.

Spirituality: Discuss the vastness of the universe. Discuss whether we are alone or whether there are other races of people in the universe!

Early Dementia: Visit a planetarium.

Late Dementia: Say or sing the old folk lullaby, "I see the moon and the moon sees me. Down through the leaves of the old oak tree."

Conversation: Ask an opinion: "Jean, do you think that wolves howl more frequently when the moon is full?" Discuss: "Would you like to go to the moon?" Share your thoughts: "Len, what does it mean to be 'over the moon' for somebody?" Tease: "Do you think the moon is really made out of cheese?"

The Basics

Establish a group of four to six *persons* (depending on the game) to play in the weekly or regularly scheduled card game and assign a staff member to provide supervision and support. Choose the game of choice: bridge, poker, gin rummy, or an old family favorite. Make sure to keep the game short to maintain concentration and reduce frustration. Enjoy a snack before or after the game. Consider playing with a partner to provide assistance to the *person* if needed.

Tip: Many people in a group can participate in this type of activity, even if they don't play cards. *Persons* can shuffle, sort poker chips, set out snacks, and just enjoy the festive atmosphere!

Variation: Partner with an individual to play solitaire.

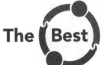

The (Best) Friends Way

Life Story: Has the *person* enjoyed playing cards? Did the *person* belong to a poker or bridge group? Has anyone won prizes at playing cards at a poker tournament or become a "Life Master" at the game of bridge? Did he or she "study the game" or just pick it up informally? Did a beloved relative teach him or her how to play certain card games?

The Arts: Enjoy the artwork on the cards.

Music: Depending on the game, some light background music might be pleasant.

Exercise: Playing cards exercises the fine motor skills.

Old Sayings: "An ace in the hole." "It's in the cards!" "Being trumped." "Royal flush." "You are such a joker!" "Poker face."

Old Skills: Shuffling and dealing cards may tap into old skills for many.

Sensory: Explore the cards—the designs and colors.

Early Dementia: Encourage the *person* to continue participating in a card group. Help the *person* adapt the game to his or her changing needs.

Late Dementia: Invite the *person* to sit with you and help you as you play a card game. Ask the *person's* help to sort the cards by suit or count them to be sure that they all are there.

Conversation: Laugh together: "Russ, you really know how to keep a poker face." Tease: "Amanda, you get very serious when you are trying to win." Reminisce: "Howard, tell me about the times you went to bridge tournaments—were they fun?" Encourage participation: "Fred, I know it's about your bedtime, but come over here and kibitz for a few minutes!" (an old-fashioned word that means looking on or watching an activity and offering comments or advice—sometimes unsolicited)

Playing Cards

Playing cards has been a pastime for many. *Persons* with dementia may enjoy maintaining this leisure activity through a regularly scheduled evening card game.

Pressed Flowers

Many of us have pressed flowers from special occasions to have as keepsakes. Pressing flowers in the evening is a low-key individual or group activity for *persons* with dementia.

The Basics

- Flowers to be pressed, picked earlier in the day from a garden or purchased
- Flower press, available at most craft stores

Together, choose which flowers you want to press and dry. Choose flowers that are not too bulky, such as daisies, asters, or cosmos, as opposed to roses and lilies. Cut the stems to about 1" to 2".

Place the flowers on the sheets of the press, filling each sheet without overlapping. Cover the flowers with a second sheet of absorbent paper. Assemble the press and tighten. Each evening, tighten the press a little more. After 2 weeks, open the flower press to find beautifully pressed and dried flowers!

Variation: Make your own press with plywood, screws, nuts and bolts, and absorbent paper, or keep it simple and press flowers in an old book or a magazine.

The 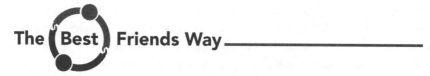 Best Friends Way

Life Story: Was the *person* a gardener or a florist? Does the *person* have a favorite flower? Did anyone press a special corsage or a flower from a wedding bouquet?

The Arts: Use the pressed flowers to create book marks or greeting cards (see Volume One, Sun Catchers, p. 89), or frame some for special gifts.

Music: Sing songs that include flowers in them: "Tiptoe Through the Tulips," "Yellow Rose of Texas."

Exercise: In summertime, when the days are long, spend time outside picking flowers after dinner.

Old Skills: Recite the poem "My Love Is Like a Red, Red Rose" (Robert Burns) or the poem about daffodils, "I Wandered Lonely as a Cloud."

Sensory: Before pressing the flowers, enjoy the sweet smell and soft feel of the petals. After the flowers are dried, discuss how the colors have changed.

Late Dementia: Take the *person* outside in a wheelchair while you pick flowers.

Conversation: Ask for help: "Marvin, would you help me tighten the flower press this evening?" Speculate together: "I wonder what the pansies will look like once they are pressed. Do you think they will hold their color?" Reminisce: "Sally, did you ever press a four-leaf clover and save it for good luck?"

The Basics

Brainstorm ideas of things that can be sorted, such as baseball cards (by team or league), playing cards (by suit), poker chips (by color), fabric pieces (to fit a quilting pattern), buttons (by type, size, or style), and nails and screws (by size or purpose). Find appropriate containers for the individuals to use to sort the item (e.g., a cupcake tin for sorting different-colored buttons).

Variation: Organize items to be used in a project the next day (e.g., materials for a crafts project, art supplies, or ingredients for a baking project).

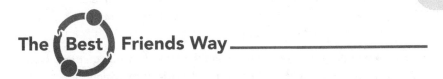

The Best Friends Way

Life Story: Identify ideas for items to sort by reviewing the life story. Be sure to connect the purpose of the activity to something in the *person's* life story. For example, sorting nails and screws may be meaningful for an individual who had a workshop at the back of his garage, or sorting fabric pieces may appeal to a quilter.

Exercise: The movement of sorting can be good exercise for the arms.

Humor: Joke about the one in the group who was very organized and the one who was not! Did anyone have a spice rack that was alphabetized?

Old Sayings: "One man's trash is another man's treasure."

Old Skills: Sorting and organizing may tap into old skills.

Sensory: Encourage the *person* to take the time to explore the materials while sorting.

Early Dementia: Invite the *person* to help you get organized. Clean out the supply closet together!

Late Dementia: Sort visually simple items, such as mixed-up checkers and dominoes.

Conversation: Ask for help: "Ella, would you help me sort out these art supplies so they'll be ready to go for tomorrow morning's class?" Explore the items: "I found an old baseball card with Babe Ruth on it. Do you remember when he played?" Work together: "Maya, these two puzzles have gotten mixed up. One puzzle is green on the back, and the other has a tan back. If you will put the green pieces in this box, then I will collect the tan ones."

Sorting with Meaning

Sorting and organizing are part of everyday life. *Persons* with dementia may enjoy sorting in the evening if they find it meaningful and are given a clear purpose for the sorting.

An ounce of prevention . . .

Make this more than busy work—offer a purpose, goal, or meaning for the activity.

Famous Pairs

Throughout history, there have been many widely known pairs, from Adam and Eve to Penn and Teller. This can be an easy evening activity as *persons* with dementia try to name as many famous pairs as they can!

The Basics

- Pictures and fun facts about famous pairs
- Flipchart
- Markers

With the group, brainstorm as many famous pairs as you can. Write them on the flipchart, and discuss those who seem to spark the most interest. Suggestions for famous pairs are as follows: Adam and Eve, Abbott and Costello, George Burns and Gracie Allen, Barnum and Bailey, Mutt and Jeff, Sears and Roebuck, Sonny and Cher, Dean Martin and Jerry Lewis, Richard Burton and Elizabeth Taylor, Lucille Ball and Desi Arnaz, Edgar Bergen and Charlie McCarthy, the Wright brothers, Simon and Garfunkel, and Fred Astaire and Ginger Rogers.

During or after the activity, show and discuss some of the pictures you've collected of famous pairs.

Variation: Give the first name in the pair and encourage *persons* to recall the second name. Watch an old movie or television show together featuring a famous pair, and share memories or laughs about the pair.

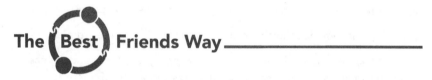

The (Best) Friends Way

Life Story: Identify famous pairs that connect with a *person's* hobbies and lifelong interests. Was anyone a twin? Did anyone ever meet a famous pair? Who in the group recalls watching Fred Astaire and Ginger Rogers dance in the movies?

The Arts: List individuals who were involved in the arts and entertaining.

Music: Identify famous pairs from the music world, such as Hank Williams, Jr. and Waylon Jennings or Johnny Cash and June Carter.

Humor: Laugh together about some of the hilarious routines of comedy's most famous pairs, such as Lucy and Desi. Watch a DVD classic comedy show.

Old Sayings: "Two of a kind." "A friend in need is a friend indeed." "Birds of a feather flock together." "It take two to tango."

Spirituality: There are several biblical pairs: Abraham and Sarah, Cain and Abel, Naomi and Ruth, Samson and Delilah, and David and Goliath.

Early Dementia: Ask for help doing the research on the famous pairs.

Late Dementia: Discuss the pictures of the pairs regardless of whether they are recognized.

Conversation: Take any pair and reminisce: "Sears and Roebuck—were they real people? Did you ever buy a refrigerator at Sears? Is that a good place to shop?" Discuss: "What are the lessons learned from David and Goliath?" Be philosophical: "Do you think that each of us has a twin somewhere in the world?"

The Basics _____

- CD player
- CDs: a variety of happy, relaxing, fun, instrumental music; possibilities include Cuban, jazz, and Irish
- Paper
- Chalk
- Colored pencils
- Markers, brushes, or paints

Announce the name or purpose of the activity to the group. Play the music and simply listen to it for a few minutes. Give a simple direction, such as, "What picture can you draw inspired by this music?" or "What kind of movement do you hear?" Spend time enjoying each creative piece inspired by the music.

Tip: You may have to take the *person's* hand and get him or her started on the activity.

Variation: Play soft, classical, or soothing music while writing poetry.

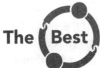

The (Best) Friends Way _____

Life Story: When possible, choose a style of music that appeals to the *person.* Perhaps he or she loves the big band sound or the Gregorian chants. Did anyone attend art school? Was anyone a skilled sketch artist, drawing pictures of people, places, or things?

Exercise: This activity stimulates fine motor skills.

Sensory: "When you close your eyes and listen to the music, what do you see?"

Spirituality: Expression through music and art can be exhilarating to the spirit.

Early Dementia: Let the *person* pick the tunes and start or stop the CD player. Ask him or her for help in setting out the supplies and planning the activity.

Late Dementia: Sit with the *person* and demonstrate drawing to the music. You may get the idea of the activity across better than when using words to try to explain the tasks.

Conversation: Celebrate together: "Look, Marge, we all drew something completely different." Compliment: "John, I like the way you painted those colorful lines while the violin music was playing." Ponder together: "Ruby, do you suppose that the great painters painted to music?" Note: "Laura, do you think you are more creative at night?"

Drawing and Painting to Music

Many artists enjoy creating to the sounds of their favorite music, such as jazz or classical. For *persons* with dementia, listening to music while drawing or painting can add a new perspective to the artwork created and fits well into a mellow evening experience.

An ounce of prevention . . .

Use music without words to avoid distraction.

Weaving

Weaving is a productive and ancient craft with rhythmic motion that can be soothing to many who like something to do with their hands. This activity adapts the age-old art of weaving to a handheld experience with simple materials that *persons* with dementia can enjoy in the evening, or anytime.

The Basics

- Corrugated cardboard 8½" × 11" (approximately)
- Yarn scraps of varying colors and textures to make the "warp" (strands of yarn that run vertically [up and down]) and the "weft" (strands of yarn that run horizontally [side to side])
- Ruler
- Scissors
- Pencil
- Straight stick the width of the piece, such as a chop stick, small twig, or narrow dowel
- Large darning needle

Make the Loom

Using the ruler, measure ¼" increments along the top and the bottom of the cardboard. Make 1" long cuts at the marks with the scissors. Make sure that the bottom cuts line up with the top. Note: This is a good activity for the Planning Group (p. 163).

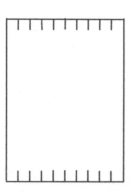

Create the Warp

Place the yarn into the first notch on the top left of the cardboard from front to back. Leave 6" hanging in front. Wrap the yarn down the back and up the front to place in the same notch. Wrap the yarn around the tab in the back, and bring it back to the front through the second notch. Take the yarn down to the bottom on the front, through the second bottom notch, up the back, and through the second top notch. Wrap the yarn around the tab in front, this time over to the third notch, and down the back, as before, all the way to the end of the cardboard to the right.

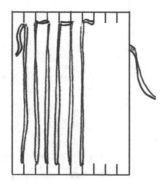

Weaving

Thread a piece of yarn through the eye of the large darning needle. From right to left at the bottom, weave over and under each successive warp yarn, all the way across. Go up to the next row. If you went under the last warp, then go over to begin the next row, weaving back to the right. Continue in this manner until there is not room at the top. When changing colors, overlap the weft threads for a few inches to secure. Be careful not to pull the weft (across) yarns too tight because it will make an hour glass shape.

Finishing

Across the back, at the top of the loom, loosen the loops between the tabs to release the tapestry from the loom. Insert a straight stick through the loops at the top and tie the threads at the bottom to form a fringe.

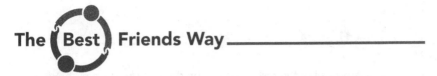

Life Story: What kinds of crafts or home decorating has the *person* done? Some like to have their hands busy all of the time. Who has visited historical sites and seen demonstrations of weaving on large floor looms? Has anyone inherited an antique loom?

The Arts: Weave an abstract design or be artistic in your color choice.

Old Skills: Needlework is an old skill to which most people can relate.

Sensory: Find as many types of yarn as possible, feel the textures, and enjoy the colors for a rich sensory experience.

Early Dementia: Invite the *person* to decide on yarn choice and patterns. *Persons* with early dementia often retain good sewing or craft skills and may continue to be part of a weaving or sewing club.

Late Dementia: Roll up or sort and organize the yarn.

Conversation: Share pride: "Otaka, just look at what we made! It is a work of art." Compliment: "Delores, I like the way you put those unusual colors together. They blend beautifully." Congratulate: "Well, team, I think this is ready for the history museum downtown. We are all accomplished fiber artists!" Wind things down: "We've had a good night's work! We've earned a good night's sleep!"

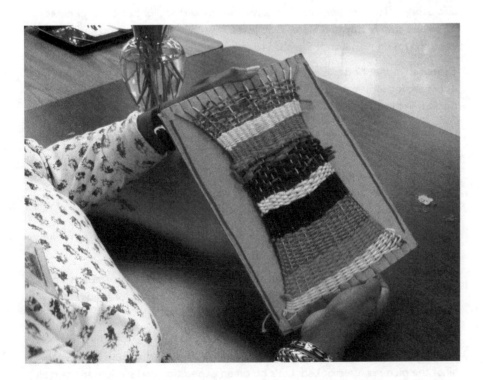

At the Close of the Day

What routines do you use to bring closure to your day? Some of us pick up the clutter from the day's activities, make a "to do" list for tomorrow, or take the dog for an evening walk. For *persons* with dementia, capping off a day can provide a helpful routine and transition them from daytime to nighttime.

The Basics

Brainstorm all of the tasks that can be done at the close of the day, such as changing notices on the bulletin board, listing tomorrow's activities, watering plants, folding clothes, drying and putting away dishes, tidying up the living area, checking fresh flower arrangements and discarding wilted or dead flowers, sending postcards or notices, copying information, arranging chairs, and cleaning the fish tank or bird aviary.

Choose to be part of this activity *persons* who like to stay busy and are not ready to "turn in" when many others are being tucked into bed.

Tip: This activity works best when the same *persons* help out each night and it becomes a routine for them.

The 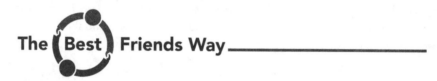 Best Friends Way

Life Story: Think of *persons* who may have worked at night or other *persons* who have always stayed up late. Who is restless early in the evening and would welcome going with a staff member to check on things?

Exercise: What better exercise after dinner than to help with checking that doors are locked, setting up the breakfast tables, or helping to sweep up some tracked-in leaves?

Old Skills: Many old skills can be tapped. Dusting the tables, stuffing envelopes, or writing a thank-you note may be appropriate for some *persons*.

Sensory: When the tasks are finished, take a few minutes to "stop and smell the roses." Sit in front of a fireplace, look at a beautiful moon, or thumb through a favorite book.

Spirituality: For those who choose to do so, stop by the chapel and sit for a while, read from a sacred text, or enjoy a prayer together.

Early Dementia: *Persons* can have certain duties that they can complete on their own, such as watering all of the potted plants, copying menus, or feeding the live-in pets.

Conversation: Tap into an old skill: "Alexa, can you help me fold these towels? You do it so well." Seek companionship: "I know I'm a bit silly, but I hate it when all of the pictures are crooked. Let's go on an expedition and straighten them all." "Stanley, will you help me make a big circle using all of these chairs?" Give a big hug: "Jessica, you are my best friend."

An ounce of prevention . . .

Some persons *may become anxious about what will be happening tomorrow. For those* persons, *keep the emphasis on the present.*

The Basics _____

Arrange to have a room open in the evening from the close of dinner to approximately 9:00 p.m. The regular activity room would be preferred if it is readily accessible. The space can be supervised by a staff member or a volunteer. Arrange some chairs for visiting or just watching. Be sure that comfortable seating is offered.

Set out a variety of activities to which *persons* might gravitate at the close of the day, such as finishing an art project; re-reading the newspaper; playing solitaire, table games, and puzzles; listening to music; or sorting and folding clothes.

Tip: It is usually not possible to staff the room at 2:00 a.m. if a *person* gets up. In those cases, take some materials from the room to create a "busy space" in the line of sight of the night shift person or next to the nurse's station.

Evening Busy Room

The old saying "early to bed and early to rise" certainly applies to many individuals. However, many *persons* with dementia are alert and active at night because of recent sleeping issues or past sleeping patterns; perhaps he or she worked the night shift. This activity creates a room just for *persons* who may be "night owls."

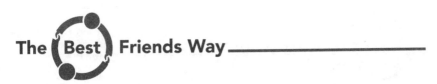

The (Best) Friends Way _____

Life Story: You may find that some *persons* grew up in families in which there were always activities in the evening for family participation. What were some of their favorite nighttime activities? Did the *person* watch "The Tonight Show" with Johnny Carson every evening before turning in (DVDs of the show are available)?

The Arts: Depending on the group on a particular night, activities can include painting a picture, creating a poem, or listening to part of an opera or a Broadway musical (see The Sound of Music, p. 198).

Exercise: A small putting strip is gentle exercise for an avid golfer.

Sensory: Many things in the room can be sensory appealing: the aroma of the fresh flowers waiting to be arranged, the sound of a favorite jazz tune in the background, or the softness of the fabric as a *person* sorts through quilting squares. Herbal teas may facilitate sleep and be a pleasurable sensory experience.

Spirituality: A *person* might like to hear a favorite religious reading, chat about his or her religious background, or look at scenes from nature or his or her favorite book of birds.

Conversation: Ask for help: "Zerelda, would you help me arrange these flowers? Our florist friend sent these cut flowers for us to enjoy." Enjoy looking through the paper together: "I always waited until the end of the day to read the paper. There are so many other things to do during the day. George, would you like to take a look with me?" Ask for help: "Would you teach me how to play solitaire? I have never played that game in my whole life."

An ounce of prevention . . .

Supervision is important for persons who have difficulty initiating an activity. Don't leave persons unattended even though they seem to be occupied.

The Sound of Music

Broadway musicals are a great source of entertainment and enjoyment for many. *Persons* may enjoy reliving the sights, sounds, and stories of the famous Rodgers and Hammerstein play and movie *The Sound of Music*. The activity can play out over several nights and can be repeated often.

The Basics

Research information on *The Sound of Music*. There is much information and trivia from fan Web sites and other sources on the Internet. Acquire pictures, clips, and music of the actors. Find a summary of the plot and song lyrics to help guide you in your discussions. Discuss trivia, such as that Mary Martin played Maria on Broadway and that Julie Andrews played her in the film.

Start the discussion by playing the opening piece, "The Sound of Music." Discuss the musical: its plot, costumes, and songs. Share historical information and tidbits, such as that the musical is based on a true story and the book *The Story of the Trapp Family Singers* by Maria Augusta von Trapp. Listen to clips of music; match it to the Broadway show.

Tip: Many DVD players have a feature that shows subtitles. This can provide instant "sing-along" lyrics to accompany the musical.

Variations: Incorporate the activity Things I Like (p. 36) with the song from *The Sound of Music*, "My Favorite Things."

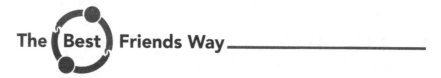

The (Best) Friends Way

Life Story: Is the *person* a fan of musical theater? Has the *person* been an actor or been involved in theater? Did the *person* enjoy traveling to New York to see Broadway shows? Does the *person* recall the first time he or she saw *The Sound of Music* movie? Has anyone traveled to Austria, where the story is set?

The Arts: Plan some art projects that involve mountains, because they play a key role in the movie.

Music: Listen and sing along to the familiar songs from the musical, such as "My Favorite Things" and "Sixteen Going on Seventeen."

Exercise: Exercise to the music.

Old Sayings: Spell out the lyrics and sing Do-Re-Mi because it is familiar and has repetition.

Sensory: Watching the rich costumes of the film can be pleasing. Look up Austrian foods on the Internet and serve something authentic to the region. Serve some fresh popcorn and enjoy the movie together.

Spirituality: Share memories of weddings prompted by Maria's spectacular wedding at the cathedral in Salzburg.

Late Dementia: Listening to the music may be comfortably familiar.

Conversation: Reminisce: "Mary, do you remember seeing *The Sound of Music* movie? Did you take your twins, Johnny and Eve?" Think of something pleasurable: "Austria is famous for its pastry; do you like desserts?"

The Basics

Discussions about art can be great fun because there is no limit to the possibilities of ideas about which to talk; there is no right or wrong way to think of art. Everyone is entitled to his or her own opinion. Look at books of collected works, such as *The Art Book* from Phaidon Press.

Begin by asking the *person* whether he or she has any thoughts to share about the piece. Listen carefully, and offer gentle encouragement to continue. Various aspects of the observations may be brought up for discussion, one at a time. Possible topics to discuss include the artwork's color, shape, content, texture, story, and feeling.

Rename the paintings. What was the artist thinking? What would you like to ask the artist about this painting? What is the most important part of the painting? What was the message that you think the artist wanted to convey by painting this? What do you like about this painting?

Variation: Borrow paintings from the public library. You can also take a "tour" of the art in your building. Some pieces could even come out of a resident's room for display and discussion (see also Mona Lisa, p. 111).

(see also Mona Lisa, p. 111).

Talking About Art

Most of us can offer a quick opinion about a painting or work of art. *Persons* with dementia can use their old skills of evaluation and offer plenty of opinions. This can be a nice one-to-one or small-group activity in the evening.

The 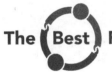 Best Friends Way

Life Story: Find out whether the *person* has had a previous interest in art. If so, then which kind of art? If the *person* has never had an interest in art, then he or she may enjoy it now or may not. Did anyone ever enjoy going to art galleries? Did someone in the group buy a painting from a street artist while on vacation in Europe?

Sensory: Bright colors, textures, patterns, and sounds stimulate the senses.

Spirituality: Study, discuss, and share the feelings that are evoked by Michelangelo's painting "Creation of Adam" in the Sistine Chapel.

Early Dementia: *Persons* can read biographies of famous artists to the others in the group.

Late Dementia: Sit together and enjoy simple, quiet conversation while holding up a painting that may be easily seen and touched.

Conversation: Give a compliment: "Alise, I would never have thought of that. You noticed how the artist used one color as a theme in the painting." Ask a simple question: "Meg, do you like bright colors?" Ponder: "Alicia, do you like modern art, or are you more traditional?" Facilitate turning in: "Mark, let's take this print you like so much to your bedroom and then I'll help you get ready for bed."

An ounce of prevention . . .

Because of the abstract nature of the ideas that can be expressed and the changes that occur in the person's brain, it is possible that a person might not understand what you are talking about and feel excluded from the conversation. For this reason, try to keep the discussion simple and light. Avoid negative topics.

Trivia with a Twist

Trivia can be used as a fun way to reminisce and experience success at the same time. This is a great low-key activity for the evening that *persons* with dementia can do in small groups or one-to-one with a caring staff member.

The Basics

Trivia can be found in books or on the Internet, or you can make up your own. (A good source is Elder Trivia; see Appendix 2.)

Using index cards, write a trivia question on one side and the answer on the other. Take turns asking each other questions, or contemplate the question together. Be sure to allow plenty of time for the *person* to answer. What's the "twist"? Giving the answer is just the first part of this activity. The twist is to discuss the answer and to give the discussion as much time as it needs. For example, if the answer to a trivia question is "meatloaf," then share favorite recipes before moving on to the next trivia question!

This activity is good for the evening because the discussion piece becomes more important than the actual trivia game. In an evening session, the group may just move at a slower pace and get through fewer questions, but actually have more "meaty" discussions!

Training Tip: Some staff members, because of their youth or because they have immigrated to the United States, may not know many answers to the trivia questions themselves. This can make it more fun for staff and *persons* with dementia to learn together.

The 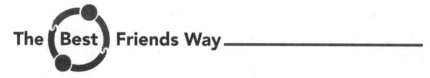 Best Friends Way

Life Story: Identify trivia that is related to the *person's* background or interest, such as sports trivia, travel trivia, movie trivia, or hometown trivia. Recognize that some have never enjoyed trivia games.

Humor: If a *person* gives a wrong answer or no one knows the answer, then joke about how trivia isn't that important. After all, it is just trivia!

Old Sayings: Although not pure trivia, it is often interesting to discuss the meaning of an old saying if it comes up. For example, the group can debate the meaning of the saying, "You can lead a horse to water, but you can't make it drink."

Old Skills: Competition is an old skill that some enjoy.

Early Dementia: Play a game of "Trivial Pursuit."

Conversation: Ask a question: "Mike, do you have a mind for trivia and small facts, or are you a big-picture guy?" Touch a life story: "Tony, I understand you know a lot about baseball statistics. What is your favorite team?" Compliment: "Gloria, you know all the answers—you are a champion!"

An ounce of prevention . . .

Watch for frustration, and be ready to assist with the answers as needed.

The Basics _____

Collect fabric and fabric scraps. Design shops or home improvement stores often have old fabric books to give away during the year. Go to the library and find books on quilting and quilting patterns. Look at quilts or quilting square pieces. List all of the patterns that you can name, such as nine patch, flower garden, and Texas star.

Discuss which patterns and fabrics you will use for a quilt. Cut out quilting pieces. Arrange them on a flannel board (see Flannel Boards, p. 182), and if the *person* is able, then assist him or her with sewing the pieces together.

Variations: Glue pieces onto poster board instead of sewing. Sort quilt pieces (see Sorting with Meaning, p. 191).

Quilting

Quilting has been a favorite pastime for many women. Quilts also play a role in family and cultural history and traditions, often serving as a historical record of a unique time or place. This activity celebrates the social connections of a quilting bee while creating something beautiful. It can be a peaceful but productive activity for *persons* with dementia during the evening.

The 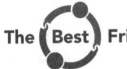 Best Friends Way _____

Life Story: Does anyone in the group recall sleeping under a homemade quilt? What types of quilts has the *person* made or owned? Ask her to show you and tell you about one of her quilts. Did anyone grow up in a region where quilt making is celebrated (e.g., Amish country, Appalachia)?

The Arts: Make a bulletin board with quilting squares and patterns.

Humor: Joke about letting your cat or dog sleep with you in bed under your quilt; is that a good idea or not?

Old Sayings: "Quilting bee." "A stitch in time saves nine." "Crazy quilt."

Old Skills: Sewing and cutting are old skills for many.

Sensory: Enjoy the stitched surface of the quilt.

Spirituality: Quilts can be left as a legacy.

Early Dementia: *Persons* may enjoy completing a quilt for a special cause or need (e.g., making baby quilts for a neonatal unit in a hospital). Many local museums have historic quilts; go to a museum for an afternoon of exploration.

Late Dementia: *Persons* may enjoy feeling fabric or the warmth of a quilt on their lap.

Conversation: Ask the group for information: "What is a quilting bee?" Make purposeful conversation: "Richard, these quilts will be wonderful to curl up under on a cold winter day." Inform: "Dr. Stock, did you know that they can make quilts out of family pictures now?" Tease: "Elmer, did you do any quilting?" Ask: "Marjorie, did you pass on your quilting skills to your daughter?"

Dried Flowers

The beauty of nature's flowers can be enjoyed year round if the flowers are dried when they are fresh. *Persons* with dementia appreciate beauty and a connection to nature even in winter. This makes a sensory-rich evening activity.

The Basics

- Fresh flowers, three or four varieties (blue, orange, and yellow flowers maintain their colors best; hydrangeas, bells of Ireland, roses, and baby's breath all dry well)
- String, approximately 7" long for each bundle

Pick fresh flowers after the morning dew has dried, or buy them at a farmer's market or store. Sort the flowers into small bundles, separating the types. Use string to tie the bundles together at the stems. Make sure that they are tied tight enough to hold all of the stems together. Hang upside down by the string in a place with no direct sunlight. Hang the flowers on a rod spaced well enough for air to pass between the bundles. Wait 4 to 5 weeks to dry completely. Arrange in baskets or vases for all to enjoy.

Variation: Dry herbs. Use the dried flowers on your festive wreath (see Festive Wreaths, p. 219).

The 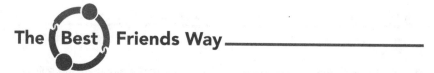 Best Friends Way

Life Story: Farmers will be able to relate to this activity; talk about whatever crops they grow and how they are preserved. Who in the group dried their wedding bouquets or corsages from a high school dance? Did anyone ever see tobacco hanging in a barn to dry?

The Arts: Use dried flowers to make note cards, bookmarks, and sun catchers (see Volume One, Sun Catchers, p. 89).

Exercise: Gathering flowers for drying can be fun and a reason for getting some physical exercise.

Humor: Joke about when you gave your sweetheart flowers to get out of trouble!

Old Skills: Picking flowers and herbs is an old skill for many that goes back to childhood.

Sensory: The dryness of the texture provides a wonderful contrast to how we are used to seeing and thinking of flowers.

Early Dementia: Grow your own flowers in raised beds, and put some aside for drying.

Late Dementia: *Persons* may enjoy touching the flowers or crushing herbs between their fingers and smelling the aroma.

Conversation: Brainstorm ideas while working: "Anna, do you think it would be a good idea to make a wreath out of these flowers when they are dried?" Ponder: "How many different types of flowers are there?" Share a concern: "Lelia, I wonder if this pretty rose aster will be the same color when it dries." Seek information: "Simon, I know you had a rose garden."

The Basics

Purchase DVDs at www.johnnycarson.com or at other Internet sellers. A few favorites are "Animal Hijinks" and "Johnny's Favorite Episodes" ($12.99 each). More information and trivia about Johnny Carson is available from multiple Web sites, including www.wikipedia.org.

Plan regular after-dinner or before-bed showings. Consider a light snack or herbal tea or decaffeinated coffee.

Adapted from Getting to Know the Life Stories of Older Adults *by Kathy Laurenhue (2007), www.healthpropress.org*

Johnny Carson

Johnny Carson was a show business legend who hosted "The Tonight Show" on NBC (now hosted by Jay Leno) for 30 years between 1962 and 1992. Many *persons* with dementia will recall Johnny, because he was virtually in their living rooms 5 nights a week. Watching "The Tonight Show" classic moments on DVD or video is a nice way to end the evening for *persons*, because it recalls an old ritual and evokes laughter and reminiscence.

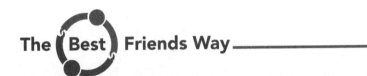 The **Best** Friends Way

Life Stories: Did the *person's* family like to watch "The Tonight Show"? Was it a ritual in the family to go to bed as soon as "The Tonight Show" was over? Was the person a "night owl," or did he or she go to bed with the chickens? Did the *person* enjoy the humor of Johnny? What was his or her favorite part of the show? Note that Johnny Carson was from Nebraska—is anyone else from the Midwest?

The Arts: Gather some pictures of Johnny in his studio, maybe one of him playing the part of Carnac the Magnificent or one of him with the many animals that visited him on his show.

Music: Play the theme song of "The Tonight Show," or sing some songs that were popular in the 1960s and 1970s. Recall some early groups, such as Sonny and Cher and the novelty act of "Tiny Tim" singing "Tiptoe Through the Tulips."

Humor: Critique the monologues, and note how sometimes it was funnier when Johnny's jokes bombed. Laugh at all of Johnny's antics with animal guests.

Old Sayings: "Here's Johnny!" "Carnac says." "How hot was it. . . ."

Sensory: The familiar pictures and sounds will stimulate many happy times watching this late-night show.

Early Dementia: Persons may fully enjoy the show and enjoy reminiscing about it.

Conversation: Laugh together: "Ani, wasn't it funny when Johnny put on that turban and pretended to be Carnac? Did you like the answers that Carnac gave?" Ask a thoughtful question: "Nelson, what was it about Johnny that endeared him to the public for all those years?" Share a common experience: "Melvin, we are two of a kind. We both nodded off long before Johnny Carson came on."

CHAPTER ELEVEN

Community Spirit

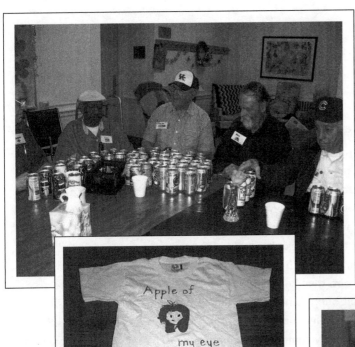

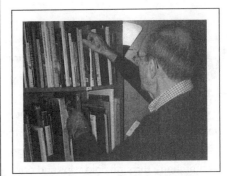

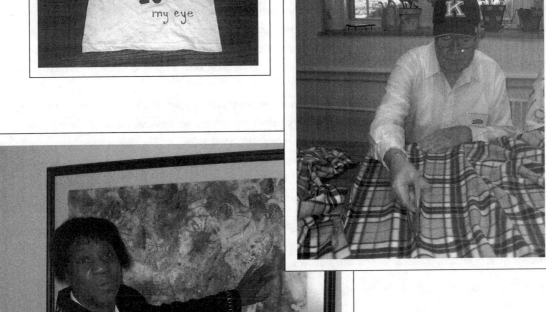

Community Spirit

Many of us have spent years working in jobs, volunteering for causes, attending concerts, going to museums, supporting a fundraising car wash, or countless other things in our community. Sadly, the *person* with dementia often becomes isolated because of his or her illness. Dementia leads to loss of driving privileges, and the *person* may have trouble initiating the activities that he or she once did for enjoyment, for work, or to help others. This can lead to sadness and depression when this active *person* gets cut off from the things that were so important to him or her.

The activities in this chapter are designed to help make it possible for *persons* to stay connected to their community through field trips and outings, as well as by doing good works for others. We call it Community Spirit! If someone is not able to travel out, then he or she can still make something to send to a local charity. We can also organize activities that bring community to the *persons* in our program.

Volunteerism still has meaning for many with dementia. A few years ago, it might have been considered outrageous to suggest that *persons* could still volunteer. Times have changed; as noted in Chapter 1, many *persons* with early-stage dementia volunteer. Carole Mulliken volunteers at her local Humane Society. Larry Sherman plays the clarinet for his friends at a day center. Later in dementia, *persons* could volunteer their efforts in other, less demanding ways, such as helping with a mailing or being in charge of handing out sheet music before a music program.

When we authentically are able to tell a *person* with dementia that an activity will help someone else, it adds meaning and relevance to something that he or she may otherwise view as frivolous. Being in the community also has considerable appeal to many *persons* who miss being active. We hope that you will use the ideas in this chapter as a starting point to help the *persons* in your care find as much meaning as possible in their lives.

We draw your attention to a few specific activities in this chapter:

Partnering with a Museum (p. 209) and Lunch Bunch (p. 216) are wonderful activities that keep a *person* in touch with past traditions and involve field trips to a museum and/or local restaurants. With the simple modifications suggested, these activities can become among your most popular.

Creating a Web Page (p. 222) has intriguing possibilities as a group project that connects the *person* to a worldwide "virtual" community.

Being an Advocate (p. 220) is an activity that was suggested by *persons* whom we interviewed for this book and involves everything from speaking at conferences and testifying before legislators (for *persons* with very early dementia) to helping write postcards for new school funding or even for Alzheimer's research.

A number of the activities involve easy but meaningful things to do for others, including Sandpaper Tote Bags (p. 217), which can be useful gifts for homeless shelters or women's shelters; Geometric Bookmarks

(p. 218), which can be a thoughtful gift for visitors, friends, or family members or a literacy program; and Festive Wreaths (p. 219), which we suggest giving to a local charity to decorate a front door.

Another activity, Mailing a Card (p. 221), is very simple but can have great significance if it is a thank-you card or a congratulatory note sent by the group to a mother who has had triplets and whom they have read about in the newspaper.

Activities with meaning, that help others, are more rewarding for *persons* and for all of us. Activities that allow us to be part of our community keep us motivated and happier. This chapter is about doing for yourself as well as doing for others.

Tips for staff training: One way to build morale and foster team spirit is to take on a community project, such as supporting the Alzheimer's Association Memory Walk, adopting an animal shelter, making blankets for a children's hospital, or doing some other worthwhile project.

CHAPTER ELEVEN ACTIVITIES

The Basics _____

Establish contact with the curator or public relations office of a museum, asking for permission to bring a small group. Go during a quiet time of the day or week, and try to arrange for a docent or museum official to talk with the group (brief them on the basics of dementia, suggesting that their comments be brief). Be sure to resolve parking issues ahead of time, and provide adequate supervision to prevent someone from getting lost. This activity lends itself to volunteer recruitment since the volunteers can also enjoy the museum experience while lending extra supervision and help.

If the museum is large, then choose a particular exhibit on which to focus to avoid fatigue. Depending on the exhibit, it can be effective to sit in front of one large painting and discuss the story or topic of the piece, the colors, the country the piece is from, the name of the artist, and the history of the piece. The group can even debate the frame!

For more on this topic, see Talking About Art, p. 199.

Variation: Check out framed paintings from the local public library for discussion.

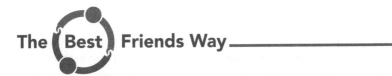

The (Best) Friends Way _____

Life Story: Discuss the *person's* particular interests in art, whether it be impressionist paintings, abstract paintings, pen-and-ink contour drawings, sculpture, or any type of art. Did someone live in a town or city that was rich with cultural attractions?

Music: "Mona Lisa" by Nat King Cole.

Exercise: Strolling through the museum incorporates exercise into the day.

Humor: Laugh together: "Did you hear that some elephants are painting with their trunks and people are paying a big price for the paintings?"

Sensory: Looking at art is visually stimulating. Go to the museum café for some goodies.

Spirituality: Many famous paintings have a religious theme. Some faith communities have collections of art to view.

Early Dementia: Partnering with a museum is a great way to stay connected to the community. A *person* can do some research on the exhibits before visiting the museum (or check that museum's Web site).

Late Dementia: Bring the art to the *person* in their care setting.

Conversation: Invite comments and opinions: "Jonah, what do you think the color of the sky in this painting tells us about the weather?" Reminisce: "Keta, did you have art classes when you were in school?" Marvel together: "Isn't it wonderful that these great paintings have been saved in their original form?"

Partnering with a Museum

Many of us enjoy the arts and appreciate a formal outing to view local and traveling exhibits. *Persons* with dementia love to be included in normal life, and a trip to a museum can be a rewarding experience.

An ounce of prevention . . .

Use common sense to ensure that persons do not touch the art inappropriately. Be cautious of potential wanderers.

209

The Culture Bus

Many of us are enriched by participating in cultural events or experiences, such as going to a music concert, visiting a museum, or going to an art gallery. The Culture Bus is an innovative way for *persons* with dementia to participate in enriching experiences, share cultural activities, enjoy outings, and make new friends.

The Basics _____

The Culture Bus is the name of an early dementia social group in Chicago. It meets every other week for a total of six outings in both spring and fall. The day (usually 10:00 a.m. to 3:00 p.m.) includes the drive to a cultural destination, such as a museum, botanical garden, planetarium, or historical society. Once there, *persons* tour the exhibit (usually with a docent), then have lunch, have a discussion, and return home. There is a charge of $55 for each outing to cover the costs of transportation, lunch fare, and applicable museum or organization entrance fees.

Submitted by Darby Morhardt, MSW, Cognitive Neurology & Alzheimer's Disease Center, Northwestern University, Chicago, IL.

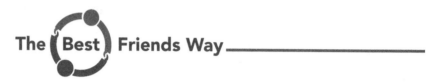

The (Best) Friends Way _____

Life Story: Has the *person* been active and participated in tours and visited cultural destinations? Identify destinations that may be of particular interest to the *person*, such as an architectural tour of the city for the architect, engineer, or construction worker.

The Arts: This activity connects all who participate with endless artistic possibilities. While you are out, notice the art in the community—monuments, nature, graffiti, and murals.

Music: Attend a concert by the local philharmonic or a smaller concert.

Old Skills: *Persons* with dementia enjoy the experience of receiving new information.

Sensory: Cultural destinations are sensory-rich experiences. Many sites have cafés where the group can pause for a snack or lunch. In good weather, the activity can also be an excuse to be out-of-doors to see a town statue or fountain or outdoor sculpture garden.

Spirituality: Darby Morhardt, who submitted this activity, explains, "In spite of shared challenges and changes in thinking and memory, participants are bound by their love for the arts, nature, history, and cultural experiences, as well as the company of one another and the continued desire for a full life in spite of dementia."

Early Dementia: This activity may be especially rewarding, offering *persons* an opportunity to maintain connections to their community or visit a favorite place.

Conversation: Ask an opinion: "Josephine, which painting do you like best?" Celebrate: "George, I am so glad that we can do this together!" Share a common interest: "Matilda, I'm so glad that you like going to a circus. Since I was a little girl, I have loved everything about a circus."

The Basics _____

Find a kit/instruction manual for creating a wooden doghouse. There are multiple sources on the Internet, but a good kit can be found at www.kitguy.com/cat_doghouse.asp.

Gather materials and develop a plan for building the doghouse. Create a work group (this is a great activity for men), and put aside time each day or week to work on the project. Have fun painting the outside with a decorative theme.

Variations: You can build other things for animals, such as a cat scratching post, a dog bed, or a birdhouse or feeder (see Volume One, Making Bird Feeders, p. 79).

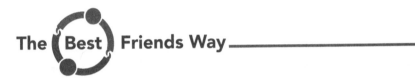

The (Best) Friends Way _____

Life Story: Has the *person* enjoyed building projects in the past? Was the *person* an architect or a carpenter? Is the *person* a dog or pet lover? Did the *person* value hard work or working with his or her hands?

The Arts: For those who may not enjoy the building aspect, invite them to decorate the inside or create a mural on one side of the doghouse.

Music: Hum "Whistle While You Work." Play fun, upbeat music in the background while you work.

Exercise: This activity is a great opportunity to maintain physical skills.

Humor: Laugh about what it means to spend time in the "doghouse."

Old Sayings: "Rome wasn't built in a day." "Many hands make light work." "You hit the nail on the head."

Old Skills: The old skills that are required for the project include hammering, sawing, sanding, and measuring.

Sensory: Listening to the pounding of the hammer or the smell of sawdust may remind a *person* of the positive atmosphere of an old workshop.

Early Dementia: Assign *persons* a particular element to coordinate, such as the painting.

Conversation: Encourage involvement: "Will you hold one end of the measuring tape for me?" Compliment: "I like the way you sanded those edges—they are so smooth!" Laugh together: "Doris, your dog has the run of the whole house. We need to build a 'people house' for your family." Joke around: "Marty, do you think poodles demand a fancier house than the average mutt?" Satisfy curiosity: "Mrs. Andersen, when you lived on the farm, did your dog sleep in the house or outside?"

Getting Out of the "Doghouse"

Creating a doghouse for "man's (or woman's) best friend" to use can be a great activity for *persons* with dementia who have enjoyed building and those who like tinkering with tools. The end product can be donated to someone in the community.

An ounce of prevention . . .

Supervision is very important in this activity to prevent injuries. Be sure to use appropriate safety equipment.

Pet Parade

Many *persons* who move to a residential facility have to give up beloved pets and mourn this loss. The Pet Parade allows *persons* with dementia to re-experience the joy of animals by inviting community pets to strut their stuff.

The Basics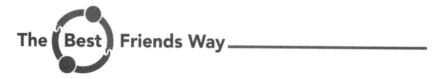

Invite staff or a local pet store to bring in a variety of pets. Make sure that all of the pets are calm natured and people oriented. If the visitor is bringing in an unusual pet, then research information about it and share it with the group. Ahead of time, work with a group to make homemade dog biscuits (see Volume One, Dog Biscuits, p. 94) as treats for the dogs that may visit.

Show each pet one at a time, announce the breed or type of animal, and share the name of the pet and any tricks that it can do. Allow plenty of time to interact with the pets.

Variation: Give a "Best in Show" ribbon or vote on your favorite animal (see I Cast My Vote for . . . , p. 174).

The (Best) Friends Way

Life Story: Does the *person* have a special pet? Has anyone participated in a pet show before? Has anyone had an unusual pet, such as an iguana or a pig? Did anyone in the group have a snake or a rat as a pet as a child (this can provide some humorous debate about the good and bad of this kind of pet!)? Did anyone have a father or other relative who was a veterinarian?

The Arts: Take pictures of *persons* with the pets.

Music: Sing, "How much is that doggie in the window?"

Exercise: Encourage the *person* to help you walk or groom a dog.

Humor: Collect look-alike pictures of people and their pets, and laugh at the resemblances. Many cartoons in magazines feature "talking animals."

Old Sayings: "Gone to the dogs." "The cat that ate the canary." "Raining cats and dogs." "A cat has nine lives."

Old Skills: It is almost impossible to have a dog or a cat greet you without evoking the old skill of patting and stroking.

Sensory: Take delight in feeling the vibrations of a cat's purr.

Early Dementia: Have the *person* be your assistant in running the pet show.

Late Dementia: Animals can often connect emotionally with *persons* without the need for words or conversation.

Conversation: Reminisce: "That is a beautiful cocker spaniel. Judy, you had a cocker spaniel as a child, right?" Ask for an opinion: "Can you teach an old dog new tricks?" Seek information: "Gerald, has your golden retriever been to obedience school?" Enjoy a friendly debate: "Ron, do you think dogs make better pets than cats?"

An ounce of prevention . . .

Be aware that some persons are frightened of animals. Orient the pet handlers about the special needs of persons with dementia.

The Basics

- Colorful cloth, netting, or voile (a lightweight, loosely woven fabric). The aroma will be stronger with a fabric that has a looser weave or that is more porous.
- Ribbon (¼" width)
- Needle and thread
- Potpourri

Cut cloth into 4" × 12" pieces. Fold in half with the right sides of the fabric together. Stitch the long sides together. Turn the bag right side out. Turn the top 2" of the bag down into the bag.

Stitch around the top of the bag 1" from the top. Repeat ½" below the first stitching, making a pathway for the ribbon. Cut a small slit in the pathway and thread a ribbon through the pathway, leaving enough ribbon to tie a bow.

Fill with potpourri. Potpourri can be made of dried flowers and herbs gathered year round by your staff and participants or can be purchased from many stores ready-made. (For more information, see Volume One, Potpourri, p. 84.)

Making Sachet Bags

Small cloth bags filled with potpourri make a sensory-rich gift for anyone who likes to tuck little sachets among the clothing in the dresser or closet. *Persons* with dementia can enjoy being a part of this rewarding project either to enjoy themselves or to give to others. Also, use them to thank volunteers or groups who come to sing or share their talents at your program.

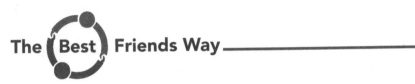

The (Best) Friends Way

Life Story: Is there a seamstress in the group? Does anyone especially like to make gifts to give to others? Who grew a garden? Did anyone grow herbs, such as sage or dill? Who in the group enjoys wearing perfume or cologne?

Old Skills: Measuring, cutting, sewing, and tying the bow all are old skills.

Sensory: The aroma of the potpourri could evoke old memories and emotions. Go outside to pick lavender, rosemary, rose petals, or other herbs or flowers from the garden.

Spirituality: Plan to have each *person* personally give the gift to someone special to him or her, thereby creating a spiritual act of sharing.

Early Dementia: *Persons* may be able to accomplish each step of this creation on his or her own or with minimal assistance.

Conversation: Enjoy the aroma together: "Nora, smell this one. It smells just like a perfume store." Reminisce: "Frederick, did you ever give your girlfriend a gardenia like this one?" Ask for help: "Ivan, would you put your finger right here while I tie this bow?" Work together: "Ruth, this rosemary has a distinct aroma. Do you like the way it smells? Did you ever cook with rosemary?"

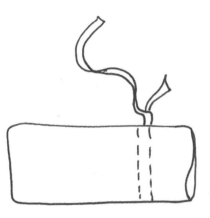

Skinny Books

Being involved in meaningful projects to help others is fulfilling to most of us. This simple project is one in which *persons* with dementia can do something meaningful for schoolchildren, perhaps even adopt a school!

The Basics

- Used or discarded books for children
- Pliers
- Scissors
- Glue
- Stapler
- Markers or paints
- Construction paper

Children who are having trouble reading are often more interested in reading a single story than reading from a book of stories. This activity takes apart old reading books to make "skinny books" that consist of one story for the children to take home to read.

Begin by taking the books apart using the pliers. Choose a story. Make a book cover that reflects the theme by using construction paper, copies of pictures from inside the book, or other sources. Use markers and paints for further decorations and to list the book's title. Staple the story securely into the cover. You may also want to stamp the book with the logo of your day or residential program (or write the name of the *persons* who created the book) on the back cover. When possible, invite the children to visit to read aloud their new book or be read to by others.

Tip: Schools often sell or give away discarded textbooks or reading books that can be used for skinny books.

Variation: Contact an elementary school in your area to ask for other ideas that your group can do for children. *Persons* can also adopt a specific class for ongoing activities.

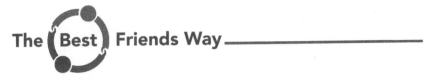

Life Story: The steps in making these books involve many old skills and trades; you can tie this activity to *persons* who are teachers or artists, *persons* who are good with tools, and "quality control" inspectors. Reminisce about favorite childhood stories or favorite books.

The Arts: The group can create its own unique design for the cover by using a theme from the book.

Old Sayings: "Book club." "Book sense." "I'm booked." "You can't judge a book by its cover."

Old Skills: Reading and helping others learn to read are familiar old skills.

Spirituality: Helping others is a core value in many of the world's religions. When a *person* is involved in helping others, he or she feels connected with his or her faith community.

Early Dementia: A *person* can coordinate the steps for most of the project. Having ongoing projects can be helpful to *persons* who may like projects to pick up at leisure times.

Late Dementia: A *person* may enjoy holding and looking through one of the books during the work time.

Conversation: Ask permission: "Fred, is this book ready to be placed in the 'ready to go' box?" Work together: "Ono, would you like to use this picture for the front cover?" Reminisce: "Goodie, did you like to read when you were a little girl in Germany?" Compliment: "Helmut, you have the knack for taking books apart."

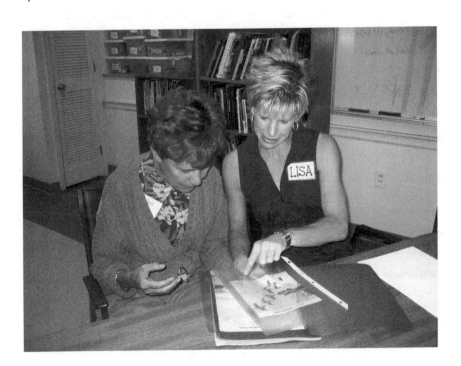

Lunch Bunch

Who hasn't enjoyed a lunch out with friends? Going out to a restaurant or local home is an important way to maintain relationships and social connectedness. This relaxed atmosphere can be helpful to *persons* with dementia, who may feel uncomfortable in some social settings.

The Basics

Choose a regular day and time for a small group, named the Lunch Bunch, to meet for lunch each week, either at a restaurant, at someone's house, or at a separate place from the regular dining room at a residential care community. For restaurants, do not go during the busiest time, and choose one that is not too noisy.

Tip: To keep the activity fresh and interesting, we suggest organizing the activity for 6 to 8 weeks, taking a break, then doing another round.

Variation: Have a Morning Coffee Club or a Dinner Society Club.

The 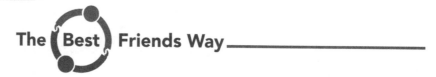 Best Friends Way

Life Story: Bring together *persons* who have similar interests or backgrounds. Did one or more in the group enjoy entertaining? Share recipes or put together a theme lunch around a *person's* past interests (e.g., British high tea, French club). Know how a *person* likes his or her coffee or tea and make note of his or her preference when serving.

The Arts: Create a lunch bunch around creative arts and get together each week to do art after enjoying a meal together.

Music: Consider listening to soft music together before or after the meal.

Exercise: After lunch, take a quick stroll together through a park.

Humor: Reminisce about culinary flops, such as the time when the cake didn't rise or you burned the roast.

Old Sayings: "The hostess with the 'most-est.'" "Life is short, eat dessert first." "Coffee klatch." "TGIF."

Old Skills: Socializing and dining with others may tap into old strengths and skills.

Sensory: The wonderful aroma of food and the joyful sounds of friendship can be very stimulating for the *person*.

Spirituality: Consider having a simple Bible study or spiritual discussion over lunch. Connecting with others is a basic need that can be met through participating in the Lunch Bunch.

Early Dementia: This activity is a great way to maintain social contacts and activities.

Conversation: Inquire: "Audrey, what is your all-time favorite food?" or "Do you like vegetables?" Have some fun: "Jeff, do you like eggplant?" Connect to his or her life story: "Here is your Earl Grey tea just like you like it, with a bit of milk" or "Here is your coffee—black and bitter." Discuss a word meaning: "Does anyone know what the word 'klatch' means when you have a 'coffee klatch'?"

An ounce of prevention . . .

Persons *usually begin to fatigue after 2 hours. Keep the activity reasonably short.*

The Basics _____

- Cloth tote bag (purchased from craft store)
- Sandpaper (medium grade)
- Plain copy paper
- Iron
- Crayons
- Cloth marker
- Fabric sealer (purchased from craft store)

Draw a design on sandpaper with crayons. Make the design bold and bright. Place the sandpaper upside down (rough side against the fabric) on the fabric bag.

Set up a safe surface for ironing. Set the iron on medium. Put a sheet of white paper underneath the fabric being ironed to prevent colors from bleeding through to the other side of the bag. Iron the back of the sandpaper to transfer the color onto the fabric. Remove the sandpaper and view your transferred design.

Use a cloth marker to outline around the shapes. Treat with a fabric sealer. Fill each bag with fresh-baked cookies or muffins, then invite some of the members of your group to help deliver them.

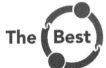

The (Best) Friends Way _____

Life Story: Did *persons* have a special bag or brief case associated with jobs? Did anyone ever backpack through Europe? What did they carry their belongings in as children? Draw pictures that connect with a lifelong hobby, such as sailing or beekeeping.

Humor: Laugh about making a "good humor" bag. Put a funny face on it.

Old Skills: Ironing, using sandpaper, and drawing exercise old skills.

Sensory: Take time to explore the different surfaces of the materials and the warm fabric bags after the transfer has been ironed.

Early Dementia: The design can be planned and detailed to cover the entire surface of the bag.

Late Dementia: Just holding the materials to get a feel for the fabric and crayons can be stimulating.

Conversation: Ask for an idea: "What kinds of things would you like to carry in this tote bag?" Reminisce: "Noah, did you carry your school books in a bag like this one?" Acknowledge a *person's* values: "Papi, you are always thinking of others. The ladies at the shelter will love this bag."

Sandpaper Tote Bags

Small tote bags can make a lovely and practical gift for residents of a homeless shelter, women's shelter, or other charitable environment. Make these to give to a chosen group. *Persons* with dementia will take pride in knowing that they have helped someone who needed a gesture of love.

An ounce of prevention . . .

Provide close supervision with the iron to prevent burns.

Geometric Bookmarks

Bookmarks are something that can make a meaningful and personal gift to a family member or a friend. They can also be donated to literacy programs. Creating a bookmark out of layered paper with a geometric design can connect a *person* with dementia to a lifelong hobby of reading and encourage others to read.

The Basics

- Cardstock, four colors
- White school glue
- Scissors
- Laminate contact paper

Measure and cut a piece of cardstock to 8½″ × 2½″ to form the basic bookmark.

Draw or trace simple geometric shapes, such as circles, squares, and triangles, on different colors of cardstock. Cut out the shapes with scissors. Overlap and layer the shapes onto the bookmark. Glue. Plan to give the bookmarks to family, friends, a school, or a literacy program.

Optional: Laminate using laminate paper or a laminating machine.

Variations: This technique may be used on placemats, scrapbooks, and greeting cards. Choose a theme for the bookmark (e.g., Hawaiian luau).

The 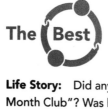 Best Friends Way

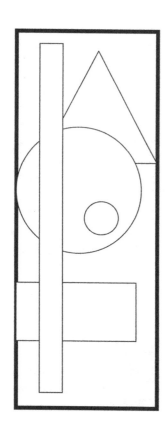

Life Story: Did anyone ever work in a bookstore or belong to the "Book-of-the-Month Club"? Was he or she an avid reader? How many *persons* like to make gifts for others? How many in the group liked to gather socially and work on a common project? Did he or she ever go to a bookstore to browse for hours and/or sit at that bookstore's café?

Music: Different colors and cut-out musical notes would make a unique design for a bookmark.

Old Sayings: "You can't judge a book by its cover." "Dog-eared." "I can read you like a book."

Sensory: Run your hand along the surface of the completed bookmark. The laminated surface feels smooth, with bumps where the paper overlaps.

Spirituality: Make a bookmark especially for use in a Bible or other religious text.

Early Dementia: Use the bookmark as a starting point to discuss a favorite book.

Late Dementia: Bright colors and simple design capture the visual interest of a *person* in late stage. Read aloud a passage from a favorite book.

Conversation: Make an observation: "Martin, I see that you are reading a mystery novel. Can you usually guess the ending?" Plan together: "These bookmarks will make great gifts for my daughter's birthday." Share a secret: "Ken, my books are all dog-eared because I mark my place by turning down the corner of the page." Share a dream: "Blanche, I hope this bookmark encourages more children to take up reading!"

The Basics _____

- Grapevine or straw wreath, may be handmade or bought
- Various items to accent the wreath, such as bows, acorns, ribbons, small toys or ornaments, or dried flowers
- Florist's wire
- Glue gun with glue sticks
- Newspapers

Lay out newspapers and warm up glue gun. Lay wreath flat on the newspapers. Arrange the accents in an interesting manner. Attach small accent items with the glue gun. Larger accents, such as pine cones, can be attached with wire wrapped around the cone. Leave a long enough length of wire to wrap and tie around the back of the wreath. Twist the wire to secure. Wrap the ribbon around the wreath in a pleasing way. Attach the bow with wire.

Variation: Make an acorn wreath by using a glue gun to attach the acorns to a straw wreath base. Work with the wreath lying flat so that no acorns will be attached to the back. Begin in the center of the wreath, placing acorns in rows all the way around until the wreath is covered with acorns. Attach ribbon or bow.

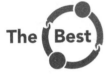

The (Best) Friends Way _____

Life Story: Use this activity for *persons* who like to stay busy. Find out whether the *person* has enjoyed growing flowers, in-home decorating, or any kind of crafts. Make a wreath with colors that have meaning to the *person*, such as school colors or national colors of a country, such as green, white, and red for Mexico.

The Arts: Make a wreath out of discarded puzzle pieces.

Humor: Make a wreath celebrating the *person's* favorite baseball team.

Sensory: The richness of texture and varieties of materials that may be used are opportunities to provide a different sensory experience by touch.

Spirituality: Creating something is a spiritual activity. The circle represents unity and wholeness.

Early Dementia: Include the *person* in the design of the wreath: choosing the theme, deciding where to put the large flowers, making the bow, and choosing colors.

Late Dementia: A *person* can give an opinion about which accents look the best on the wreath.

Conversation: Ask for a long-term memory: "Paulette, did you swing on a grapevine when you were little?" Compliment: "Tonya, have you always been good with your hands?" Reminisce: "Did your wife, Ellen, ever hang wreaths on the front door to celebrate a special occasion or season?" Encourage involvement: "John, as an engineer, can you help us design the best hook to make sure that it stays put on the front door and doesn't fall off?"

Festive Wreaths

Create a wreath to commemorate a season or holiday. For *persons* with dementia, a wreath communicates a festive, nostalgic air of celebration. Give the wreath to a family member or a friend, a special staff member, or a local charity to decorate its front door.

An ounce of prevention . . .

Glue guns get extremely hot. It can be a trick to hold the piece down well enough for it to adhere and not get any glue on the fingers. Supervise well.

Being an Advocate

In many ways, all of us are advocates from time to time, whether for ourselves (asking for a pay raise, negotiating a better price on a home improvement) or for others (opposing a zoning change in your community or writing a letter to Congress for medical research). *Persons* with dementia may still find advocacy meaningful, be it at a local or a national level.

The Basics

Use *USA Today* (see USA Today, p. 43) or a local paper to read the news with a small group of *persons* in your program. Single out a specific issue or two that would lend themselves to an advocacy effort (choose something without significant controversy, such as supporting a local charitable effort to build a hospital that supports research, or conducting a holiday toy drive).

Pass out postcards and pens, then encourage *persons* to write a note of support for the project you have chosen.

Variations:

1. Attend an Alzheimer's Association Memory Walk as a group or other worthy charitable events.
2. Create a petition (again on a noncontroversial subject) and encourage *persons* in the group to sign it.
3. Get involved in advocacy related to aging and dementia by writing Congress for more research funding or supporting the growth of local services.

The (Best) Friends Way

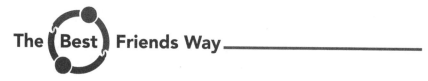

Life Story: Have any *persons* been active as advocates (e.g., written letters, made speeches, demonstrated)? Have any *persons* served on city councils, on school boards, or in state government? Who advocated for a new swimming pool, park, library, or a new school for their community?

The Arts: Making posters or creating fliers or even a bulletin board on a theme such as supporting the environment can be a part of an advocacy program.

Music: An advocacy day or activity presents an opportunity to listen to patriotic music ("God Bless America" or "America the Beautiful").

Old Sayings: "One man, one vote" (or joke that it should be "one woman, two votes!").

Old Skills: *Persons* retain the old skill of signing their name far into dementia and often are pleased to be asked to add their name to support a cause.

Early Dementia: *Persons* may enjoy being on local advocacy committees for the Alzheimer's Association, speaking at local hearings, writing letters to the editor, supporting public awareness or media efforts.

Conversation: Compliment: "Judge, you must be very proud that you were a big supporter of the park along the river. Just think how many families, friends, and out-of-town visitors are enjoying that lovely space." Be thoughtful together: "Aren't we grateful for all those people who have worked hard to make life better for all of us?"

The Basics ─────────────

- Miscellaneous occasion or postcards; blank cards to write notes
- Pencils or pens
- Addresses
- Stamps

Discuss special occasions that call for a greeting card. Help *persons* choose one to send. Encourage them to write a greeting and sign their name to the cards. Prepare the cards for mailing by writing the address on the envelope and placing a stamp on it. Together, walk to the mailbox to mail the card or take a trip to the post office.

Variation: Read through local newspapers and identify individuals in the community who have won awards or been recognized for special achievements; write a collective card to them.

Submitted by Amy Wise, Assistant Health Care Director, Elmcroft of Halls, Knoxville, TN.

The (Best) Friends Way ─────────────

Life Story: Did the *person* study handwriting in school, learning how to make cursive letters? Was he or she someone who always remembered family birthdays, anniversaries, and other occasions? Did he or she send lots of postcards while on vacation? Did he or she ever have business letterhead or embossed stationery?

The Arts: Make the greeting card (see Volume One, Creating One-of-a-Kind Greeting Cards, p. 77).

Exercise: Walking to the mailbox incorporates physical activity into each day.

Humor: Write funny jokes or sayings in the cards, such as "Happy 39th Birthday—Again!" Keep on hand a supply of humorous cards.

Old Sayings: Many greeting cards have simple but sweet poems or sayings. Take time to read them aloud and discuss their meaning.

Old Skills: Sorting through old letters and cards may be an old skill for many.

Sensory: Enjoy a cup of tea while the group is gathered and preparing the cards.

Early Dementia: This activity is a great way to maintain social connections and express one's thoughts and best wishes for another.

Conversation: Share a thought: "Alicia, Henrietta's daughter is having her 40th birthday. Do you think that life begins at 40?" Compliment: "Walter, have you always had such beautiful handwriting? Did you study penmanship? It is so easy to read." Ponder together: "Inez, look at this. Molly's great-grandson and his wife are having twins. Can you imagine taking care of two babies at once?"

Mailing a Card

Writing a note or sending a greeting card or a postcard can represent a time to pause and think about friends and family. Mailing a card involves the *person* with dementia in an activity that incorporates everyday activities that were performed in the past.

An ounce of prevention . . .

Visual–spatial problems and loss of language skills can come with dementia and interfere with a person's ability to write.

Creating a Web Page

The use of the World Wide Web is not, contrary to conventional wisdom, the sole domain of young people. More and more older adults have e-mail, use Web sites, and surf the Web regularly. Creating a Web page or Web site for your program is a wonderful group project and allows the group to share news and photographs, as well as facilitate e-mail. It also helps the *person* with dementia feel part of the worldwide community!

An ounce of prevention . . .

It is possible to establish passwords that would control access to the Web site that could be given out to family members, but it is important to obtain appropriate written permission from the person or from his or her responsible party to display personal information and images.

The Basics _____

Use a free or low-cost Internet service provider to create a Web page or Web site for your program using the basic software. Involve *persons* with dementia as much as possible in design decisions, entering information, proofreading pages, or other tasks.

Share program news, activity calendars, trivia, stories, and photographs with your Web visitors. Other topics could include favorite recipes. The site can also be designed to allow family members to e-mail loved ones.

This makes a great intergenerational activity, because many young people are Web savvy and would enjoy helping an older friend or relative with the project.

Variations: Help an individual in your program create his or her personal Web page or Web site.

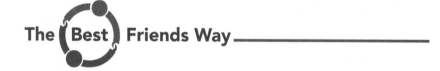

The (Best) Friends Way _____

Life Story: Who has been fascinated with the Web from the time it appeared several years ago? How many *persons* are computer literate? Who has been a part of a chat group on the Web? Does anyone like to spend time surfing the Web? Who would like to try something new?

The Arts: Someone will need to create the artwork or logo for the Web page. Also, pictures will need to be chosen to support some of the text.

Spirituality: Many sites that support spiritual life, such as arts-related sites, travel-related sites, and sites that are devoted to charitable causes, are available on the Web. Many sites also offer information about religious practices.

Early Dementia: Some *persons* undoubtedly will already be experts in creating a Web page and can lead the way in helping to design it and get it up and going. Most of the younger *persons* who are in the programs now are very familiar with the Internet.

Conversation: Reminisce: "It is difficult to think of the time before the computer. Larry, don't you wonder how we managed without e-mail?" Encourage conversation: "Lois, did you have a computer when you were growing up?" Ponder the marvel of all of our technology: "Julian, do you know how a message gets from your computer to the computer of your friend in India?" Reminisce: "Beulah, do you still have your old typewriter?"

CHAPTER TWELVE

Conclusion

Some of the best people in the world work in dementia care. Earnest, caring, bright, enthusiastic, and fun, they work hard, find success and satisfaction, but at the same time tell us that they feel a lot of pressure, carrying "the whole world on our shoulders." How can activity directors, administrators, nurses, certified nurse assistants, or other staff members go about building a better program given their already heavy workload? How can new ideas get implemented? Here are some recommendations.

Start with an easy step, one that is not overwhelming. Take one activity in this book and do it once a week. Choose something easy, such as Daily Intentional Walking (p. 69). Congratulations, you have just added 52 hours a year of quality to your dementia care program. Keep going. Add another simple program to the calendar—how about An Old-Fashioned Tea (p. 152) or Happy Hour (p. 187)? Do one of these once a week and it is another 52 hours a year of great activities.

Can your program afford a 75-cent expenditure? Go out and buy a copy of *USA Today* (p. 43). Staff can map hometowns of *persons* in your program on the newspaper's oversized weather map, study state-by-state news, review sports results of a *person's* favorite team, or admire new fashions or new cars in large, colorful advertisements. When you are done, save a few pages to make a festive paper hat—celebrate that you have just added another 52 hours a year of quality to your program for less than $1.00 a week.

Do you enjoy learning? Announce to your team that you have created "Best Friends University." By taking to heart the concepts in Chapter 6, "Adult Education," you can easily create a 1-hour class to teach once a week. The trivia and group exercises are growth opportunities for *persons* and for staff. Let's all get smarter this year as we add another 52 hours a year of excellence to our programs.

Are you a bit of a gambler? Throw a dart. By that, we mean open up this activity book (or Volume One) once or twice a month to a random page and do the activity the following week. This keeps it fresh and fun; maybe you will be learning about Maple Harvest (p. 109), the Northern Lights (p. 110), or Touring Mexico (p. 101). Again, you have added 52 hours a year of excellence to your program.

Change is sometimes slow in coming, but if just 10 people with dementia in your program do five of the above activities weekly for a year, you have enriched the lives of *persons* with dementia (and the lives of everyone participating, including staff, volunteers, and families) by 2,600 hours of Best Friends activities.

Change can also come in minutes instead of hours. The activities in Chapter 2, "Celebrating the Moment," take almost no preparation and no budget. Through role playing and training, teach your staff to celebrate the moment. When they take just 30 seconds to be a bit less task oriented and to be a bit more *person* centered, care improves dramatically. Watch This! (p. 19) and Prompt Me with Dignity (p. 27) are two examples of everyday activities that, when done over time, will add hundreds of hours of excellence to your dementia program.

We are off to a great start. Now how do you get some help? We often hear that activities profession-als have trouble getting other staff to do activities. One tip for you is to take some time (we know that is hard!) to orient them better on activities. Take an activity such as Fun with Scarves (p. 171) and turn it into a staff in-service session. At first they may grumble, but then they will have a lot of fun and learn some valuable lessons about social engagement, and how easy it can be to bring a smile to others. We all learn new information best by doing.

Let's borrow an idea from the retail and restaurant industries. Many stores have quick "stand up" meetings at the beginning of the shift. Motivated managers will sometimes lay down a daily challenge. "Today is red-tie day. For every red tie you sell, you get a $5 bonus in your paycheck!" Restaurants some-times do the same thing: "Move the pumpkin cheesecake. You get a raffle ticket for every piece you sell, and the winner tonight gets a $50 gift certificate."

Can you develop a "cheesecake moment" at your program? Hand out trivia questions on cards to staff at the beginning of a shift. If a staff member picks a resident, does the trivia, writes down his or her name and the resident's name on the card, and puts it in a box by the end of the day, then he or she is eli-gible for a raffle prize.

One dementia unit had an old-fashioned clothesline outside that was meant to evoke memories of home. Nice idea, but no one ever used it! The unit director brought in wooden clothespins one sunny day. She told the staff, "Write your name on the clothespin. Find a resident today, and together pin up an item of clothing on the clothesline. At the end of the day, I'll take down the clothes and clothespins, put the pins in a hat, draw a name, and present some prizes."

Staff pay attention when they are well oriented, encouraged, given clear directions, and rewarded!

Richard Taylor, a *person* with early dementia featured in the Introduction, says it well when he asks all of us to "enable me, re-enable me, and for God's sake, don't disable me!" An excellent activity program can "enable" *persons* with dementia to be at their best. It can also help us *be* a Best Friend to a *person* with dementia, and perhaps to *make* a Best Friend at the same time.

Good luck creating your Best Friends activity program. Please visit us on the Web at www .bestfriendsapproach.com and share with us your successes. We plan to post "best practices" or success-ful activities on our Web site on a regular basis. We would love to hear how you are doing.

Collage Materials

Almost anything can be used for a collage, as long as it is clean and lightweight (so it can be easily glued to the background).

aluminum foil	junk mail	plastic spoons
beads	keys	postcards
bells	lace	puzzle pieces
bottle tops	leaves	ribbon
broken jewelry	magazines	sequins
broken toys	make-up brushes	shells
bubble wrap	meat trays	shoelaces
business cards	nuts & bolts	silk flowers
chewing gum wrappers	nutshells	small gift boxes
clothes pins	old art projects	small milk cartons
coffee filters	old buttons	sponges
colored paper	old calendars	stickers
corks	old cards	sticks
cotton balls	old compact discs	stones
dried beans	old movie tickets	tags
dried flowers	old phone book pages	travel brochures
egg cartons	old stamps	tree bark
eggshells	paper doilies	twine
empty ribbon holders	pencils	used envelopes
feathers	photographs	used gift wrap
greeting cards	picture frames	wallpaper
ice pop sticks	pieces of wire screen	wire
jar lids	pipe cleaners	yarn

Resources for Activities Professionals

Suggested Books

Alzheimer's Association. (1995). *Activity programming for persons with dementia. A Sourcebook.* Chicago: Author.

Bell, V., & Troxel, D. (1996). *The Best Friends approach to Alzheimer's care.* Baltimore: Health Professions Press.

Bell, V., & Troxel, D. (2001). *A dignified life: The Best Friends approach to Alzheimer's care.* Deerfield Beach, FL: Health Communications, Inc.

Bell, V., & Troxel, D. (2002). *The Best Friends staff book: Building a culture of care in Alzheimer's programs.* Baltimore: Health Professions Press.

Bell, V., Troxel, D., Cox, T., & Hamon, R. (2004). *The Best Friends book of Alzheimer's activities* (Vol. 1). Baltimore: Health Professions Press.

Barrick, A. L., Rader, J., & Hoeffer, B. (2001). *Bathing without a battle: Personal care of individuals with dementia.* New York: Springer Publishing Company.

Boden, C. (1998). *Who will I be when I die?* New York: HarperCollins.

Bowlby Sifton, C. (2004). *Navigating the Alzheimer's journey—A compass for caregiving.* Baltimore: Health Professions Press.

Bryden, C. (2005). *Dancing with dementia.* London: Jessica Kingsley.

Dowling, J. R. (1995). *Keeping busy: A handbook of activities for persons with dementia.* Baltimore: Johns Hopkins University Press.

Fister, B., & Valentine, S. (2006). *Field of themes: 100 activities for our senior friends.* New York: Brookdale Foundation (www.brookdalefoundation.org).

Gibson, F. (2004). *The past in the present: Using reminiscence in health and social care.* Baltimore: Health Professions Press.

Hellen, C. (1998). *Alzheimer's disease: Activity-focused care* (2nd ed.). Boston: Butterworth-Heinemann.

Jenny, S., & Oropeza, M. (1993). *Memories in the making: A program of creative art expression for Alzheimer's patients.* Irvine, CA: Phoenix Press.

Kuhn, D. (2003). *Alzheimer's early stages: First steps for families, friends, and caregivers.* Alameda, CA: Hunter House.

Larsen, B. (2006). *Movement with meaning: A multisensory program for individuals with early-stage Alzheimer's disease.* Baltimore: Health Professions Press.

Laurenhue, K. (2007). *Getting to know the life stories of older adults: Activities for building relationships.* Baltimore: Health Professions Press.

Lee, J. (2003). *Just love me: My life turned upside down by Alzheimer's.* Lafayette, IN: Purdue University Press.

Levine Madori, L. (2005). *Therapeutic thematic arts programming for older adults.* Baltimore: Health Professions Press.

McKillop, J. (2003). *Opening shutters—opening minds* (available from the Iris Murdoch Centre at Stirling University, www.dementia.stir.ac.uk/publications.htm).

Merriam-Webster. (1999). *Merriam-Webster's rhyming dictionary.* New York: Author.

Mobley, T. (2004). *Young hope.* Hazelwood, MO: Emerald Falcon Press.

Mobley, T., & Mobley, A. (2006). *I remember when.* Hazelwood, MO: Emerald Falcon Press.

Schneider, C. (2006). *Don't bury me.* Bloomington, IN: AuthorHouse (www.authorhouse.com).

Steven, T. (2002). *It is not promised: A collection of poems.* Santa Barbara, CA: Tap Steven Books (available from California Central Coast Alzheimer's Association, www.centralcoastalz.org).

Taylor, R. (2007). *Alzheimer's from the inside out.* Baltimore: Health Professions Press.

Wells, S. (1998). *Horticultural therapy and the older adult population.* Binghamton, NY: Hawarth Press.

Zgola, J., & Bordillon, G. (2001). *Bon appetit! The joy of dining in long-term care.* Baltimore: Health Professions Press.

Recommended Web Sites

Activity Connection, www.activityconnection.com: This subscription-based Web site has excellent materials and ideas about activities.

Alternative Solutions in Long Term Care, www.activitytherapy.com: This Web site is a helpful gateway for activity professionals, with a rich listing of resource materials, holidays, bulletin board ideas, and other materials.

American Horticultural Therapy Association, www.ahta.org: This Web site is for those who are interested in the therapeutic benefits of gardening; it includes publications and research as well as upcoming events and meetings.

Best Friends Approach, www.bestfriendsapproach.com: The official Web site of the Best Friends model of care, with handouts available for free downloading and updates on the authors' work.

Dementia Advocacy and Support Network International (DASNI), www.dasninternational.org: Influential and informative Web site created by and offered for *persons* with early dementia; includes opportunities for networking and resources for early-onset and early-stage *persons* with dementia.

Mary's Place, www.angelfire.com/ok4/mari5113/index.html: Informative site by Mary Lockhart, a *person* with early dementia featured in Chapter 1 of this book.

National Alzheimer's Association, www.alz.org: This Web site has links to local member chapters and the well-regarded Green-Field Library at its Chicago office.

National Center for Creative Aging, www.creativeaging.org: This is the Web site for an organization and clearinghouse for professionals who are interested in creativity and aging.

Therapeutic Recreation Directory, www.recreationtherapy.com: This Web site contains resources for recreation therapists, therapeutic recreation specialists, creative arts therapists, activity therapists, activity directors, and professionals in other disciplines.

Wikipedia, www.wikipedia.org: A worldwide collaborative online encyclopedia and a great source of history and trivia on almost any topic.

Wiser Now, Inc., www.wisernow.com: Useful site by Kathy Laurenhue, with information about activities and program development.

Journals

Activities Directors' Quarterly for Alzheimer's & Other Dementia Patients
www.alzheimersjournal.com/pn08000.html

Alzheimer's Care Today
Telephone: 800-638-3030 or 301-223-2300

American Journal of Recreation Therapy
www.pnpco.com/pn10000.html

Creative Forecasting
www.creativeforecasting.com

Vendors

The Alzheimer's Store: An Ageless Design Company, www.alzstore.com: Online store owned by the well-regarded Mark and Ellen Warner; great resource for a variety of activity products, publications, and other products for family and professional caregivers.

Bi-Folkal Productions, Inc., www.bifolkal.org: This company provides program ideas and resources for activity programs.

Elder Games, www.ncoa.org/content.cfm?sectionID=30: Nonprofit service of the National Council on Aging, with many trivia and game resources.

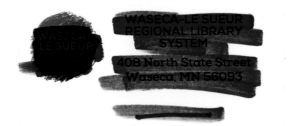